CHOLESTEROL, ATHEROSCLEROSIS AND CORONARY DISEASE IN THE UK, 1950–2000

The transcript of a Witness Seminar held by the Wellcome Trust Centre for the History of Medicine at UCL, London, on 8 March 2005

Edited by L A Reynolds and E M Tansey

Volume 27 2006

[redacted]

First published by the Wellcome Trust Centre
for the History of Medicine at UCL, 2006

The Wellcome Trust Centre for the History of Medicine
at UCL is funded by the Wellcome Trust, which is
a registered charity, no. 210183.

ISBN 0 85484 107 5
ISBN 978 085484 107 3

All volumes are freely available online following the links to Publications/Wellcome Witnesses at www.ucl.ac.uk/histmed

Technology Transfer in Britain: The case of monoclonal antibodies; Self and Non-Self: A history of autoimmunity; Endogenous Opiates; The Committee on Safety of Drugs • Making the Human Body Transparent: The impact of NMR and MRI; Research in General Practice; Drugs in Psychiatric Practice; The MRC Common Cold Unit • Early Heart Transplant Surgery in the UK • Haemophilia: Recent history of clinical management • Looking at the Unborn: Historical aspects of obstetric ultrasound • Post Penicillin Antibiotics: From acceptance to resistance? • Clinical Research in Britain, 1950–1980 • Intestinal Absorption • Origins of Neonatal Intensive Care in the UK • British Contributions to Medical Research and Education in Africa after the Second World War • Childhood Asthma and Beyond • Maternal Care • Population-based Research in South Wales: The MRC Pneumoconiosis Research Unit and the MRC Epidemiology Unit • Peptic Ulcer: Rise and fall • Leukaemia • The MRC Applied Psychology Unit • Genetic Testing • Foot and Mouth Disease: The 1967 outbreak and its aftermath • Environmental Toxicology: The legacy of *Silent Spring* • Cystic Fibrosis • Innovation in Pain Management • The Rhesus Factor and Disease Prevention • The Recent History of Platelets in Thrombosis and Other Disorders • Short-course Chemotherapy for Tuberculosis • Prenatal Corticosteroids for Reducing Morbidity and Mortality after Preterm Birth • Public Health in the 1980s and 1990s: Decline and rise? • Cholesterol, Atherosclerosis and Coronary Disease in the UK, 1950–2000

CONTENTS

ILLUSTRATIONS AND CREDITS

WITNESS SEMINARS: MEETINGS AND PUBLICATIONS[1]

In 1990 the Wellcome Trust created a History of Twentieth Century Medicine Group, associated with the Academic Unit of the Wellcome Institute for the History of Medicine, to bring together clinicians, scientists, historians and others interested in contemporary medical history. Among a number of other initiatives the format of Witness Seminars, used by the Institute of Contemporary British History to address issues of recent political history, was adopted, to promote interaction between these different groups, to emphasize the potential benefits of working jointly, and to encourage the creation and deposit of archival sources for present and future use. In June 1999 the Governors of the Wellcome Trust decided that it would be appropriate for the Academic Unit to enjoy a more formal academic affiliation and turned the Unit into the Wellcome Trust Centre for the History of Medicine at UCL from 1 October 2000. The Wellcome Trust continues to fund the Witness Seminar programme via its support for the Wellcome Trust Centre.

The Witness Seminar is a particularly specialized form of oral history, where several people associated with a particular set of circumstances or events are invited to come together to discuss, debate, and agree or disagree about their memories. To date, the History of Twentieth Century Medicine Group has held more than 40 such meetings, most of which have been published, as listed on pages xi–xix.

Subjects are usually proposed by, or through, members of the Programme Committee of the Group, which includes professional historians of medicine, practising scientists and clinicians, and once an appropriate topic has been agreed, suitable participants are identified and invited. This inevitably leads to further contacts, and more suggestions of people to invite. As the organization of the meeting progresses, a flexible outline plan for the meeting is devised, usually with assistance from the meeting's chairman, and some participants are invited to 'start the ball rolling' on particular themes, by speaking for a short period to initiate and stimulate further discussion.

[1] The following text also appears in the 'Introduction' to recent volumes of *Wellcome Witnesses to Twentieth Century Medicine* published by the Wellcome Trust and the Wellcome Trust Centre for the History of Medicine at UCL.

Each meeting is fully recorded, the tapes are transcribed and the unedited transcript is immediately sent to every participant. Each is asked to check his or her own contributions and to provide brief biographical details. The editors turn the transcript into readable text, and participants' minor corrections and comments are incorporated into that text, while biographical and bibliographical details are added as footnotes, as are more substantial comments and additional material provided by participants. The final scripts are then sent to every contributor, accompanied by forms assigning copyright to the Wellcome Trust. Copies of all additional correspondence received during the editorial process are deposited with the records of each meeting in Archives and Manuscripts, Wellcome Library, London.

As with all our meetings, we hope that even if the precise details of some of the technical sections are not clear to the non-specialist, the sense and significance of the events will be understandable. Our aim is for the volumes that emerge from these meetings to inform those with a general interest in the history of modern medicine and medical science; to provide historians with new insights, fresh material for study, and further themes for research; and to emphasize to the participants that events of the recent past, of their own working lives, are of proper and necessary concern to historians.

ACKNOWLEDGEMENTS

'Cholesterol' was suggested as a suitable topic for a Witness Seminar by Professor Michael Oliver, who assisted us in planning the meeting. We are very grateful to him for his input and his excellent chairing of the occasion. We are particularly grateful to Dr Nick Myant for writing such a useful introduction to these published proceedings. Our additional thanks go to Professor Gerry Shaper and Dr Jonathan Tobert for their help preparing the appendices for publication; Dr Paul Miller, who read through earlier drafts of the transcript, and offered helpful comments and advice. We thank the contributors for help with the glossary; Professors Michael Oliver and Chris Packard for help with table 2; Professors Jerry Morris, Michael Oliver, Dr W F M Fulton and Professors Gilbert Thompson and Neville Woolf for additional help with photographs; Ms Rocio Lale-Montes for editorial assistance with the introduction; and Charles C Thomas Publisher, Ltd, Springfield, Illinois, and the Nutrition Society for permission to reproduce images in this volume.

As with all our meetings, we depend a great deal on our colleagues at the Wellcome Trust to ensure their smooth running: the Audiovisual Department, and the Medical Photographic Library and Mrs Tracy Tillotson of the Wellcome Library; Akio Morishima, who has supervised the design and production of this volume; our indexer, Liza Furnival; and our readers, Ms Lucy Moore, Ms Fiona Plowman and Mr Simon Reynolds. Mrs Jaqui Carter is our transcriber, and Mrs Wendy Kutner and Dr Daphne Christie assist us in running the meetings. Finally, we thank the Wellcome Trust for supporting this programme.

Tilli Tansey

Lois Reynolds

Wellcome Trust Centre for the History of Medicine at UCL

HISTORY OF TWENTIETH CENTURY MEDICINE WITNESS SEMINARS, 1993–2006

1993 **Monoclonal antibodies**
Organizers: Dr E M Tansey and Dr Peter Catterall

1994 **The early history of renal transplantation**
Organizer: Dr Stephen Lock

Pneumoconiosis of coal workers
Organizer: Dr E M Tansey

1995 **Self and non-self: A history of autoimmunity**
Organizers: Sir Christopher Booth and Dr E M Tansey

Ashes to ashes: The history of smoking and health
Organizers: Dr Stephen Lock and Dr E M Tansey

Oral contraceptives
Organizers: Dr Lara Marks and Dr E M Tansey

Endogenous opiates
Organizer: Dr E M Tansey

1996 **Committee on Safety of Drugs**
Organizers: Dr Stephen Lock and Dr E M Tansey

Making the body more transparent: The impact of nuclear magnetic resonance and magnetic resonance imaging
Organizer: Sir Christopher Booth

1997 **Research in general practice**
Organizers: Dr Ian Tait and Dr E M Tansey

Drugs in psychiatric practice
Organizers: Dr David Healy and Dr E M Tansey

The MRC Common Cold Unit
Organizers: Dr David Tyrrell and Dr E M Tansey

The first heart transplant in the UK
Organizer: Professor Tom Treasure

1998 **Haemophilia: Recent history of clinical management**
Organizers: Professor Christine Lee and Dr E M Tansey

Obstetric ultrasound: Historical perspectives
Organizers: Dr Malcolm Nicolson, Mr John Fleming and Dr E M Tansey

Post penicillin antibiotics
Organizers: Dr Robert Bud and Dr E M Tansey

Clinical research in Britain, 1950–1980
Organizers: Dr David Gordon and Dr E M Tansey

1999 **Intestinal absorption**
Organizers: Sir Christopher Booth and Dr E M Tansey

The MRC Epidemiology Unit (South Wales)
Organizers: Dr Andy Ness and Dr E M Tansey

Neonatal intensive care
Organizers: Professor Osmund Reynolds and Dr E M Tansey

British contributions to medicine in Africa after the Second World War
Organizers: Dr Mary Dobson, Dr Maureen Malowany, Dr Gordon Cook and Dr E M Tansey

2000 **Childhood asthma, and beyond**
Organizers: Dr Chris O'Callaghan and Dr Daphne Christie

Peptic ulcer: Rise and fall
Organizers: Sir Christopher Booth, Professor Roy Pounder and Dr E M Tansey

Maternal care
Organizers: Dr Irvine Loudon and Dr Daphne Christie

2001 **Leukaemia**
Organizers: Professor Sir David Weatherall, Professor John Goldman, Sir Christopher Booth and Dr Daphne Christie

The MRC Applied Psychology Unit
Organizers: Dr Geoff Bunn and Dr Daphne Christie

Genetic testing
Organizers: Professor Doris Zallen and Dr Daphne Christie

Foot and mouth disease: The 1967 outbreak and its aftermath
Organizers: Dr Abigail Woods, Dr Daphne Christie and Dr David Aickin

2002 **Environmental toxicology: The legacy of *Silent Spring***
Organizers: Dr Robert Flanagan and Dr Daphne Christie

Cystic fibrosis
Organizers: Dr James Littlewood and Dr Daphne Christie

Innovation in pain management
Organizers: Professor David Clark and Dr Daphne Christie

2003 **Thrombolysis**
Organizers: Mr Robert Arnott and Dr Daphne Christie

Beyond the asylum: Anti-psychiatry and care in the community
Organizers: Dr Mark Jackson and Dr Daphne Christie

The Rhesus factor and disease prevention
Organizers: Professor Doris Zallen and Dr Daphne Christie

Platelets in thrombosis and other disorders
Organizers: Professor Gustav Born and Dr Daphne Christie

2004 **Short-course chemotherapy for tuberculosis**
Organizers: Dr Owen McCarthy and Dr Daphne Christie

Prenatal corticosteroids for reducing morbidity and mortality associated with preterm birth
Organizers: Sir Iain Chalmers and Dr Daphne Christie

Public health in the 1980s and 1990s: Decline and rise?
Organizers: Professor Virginia Berridge, Dr Niki Ellis and Dr Daphne Christie

2005 **The history of cholesterol, atherosclerosis and coronary disease, 1950–2000**
Organizers: Professor Michael Oliver and Dr Daphne Christie

Development of physics applied to medicine in the UK, 1945–90
Organizers: Professor John Clifton and Dr Daphne Christie

2006 **The early development of total hip replacement**
Advisers: Dr Krishna Kunzru and Dr Francis Neary

The discovery, use and impact of platinum salts as chemotherapy agents for cancer
Advisers: Professor Paul Andrews and Dr Anthony Woods

Medical ethics education in Britain, 1963–93
Adviser: Dr Michael Barr

Superbugs and superdrugs: The history of MRSA
Adviser: Professor Gordon Stewart

PUBLISHED MEETINGS

'...Few books are so intellectually stimulating or uplifting'.
Journal of the Royal Society of Medicine (1999) **92:** 206–8,
review of vols 1 and 2

'...This is oral history at its best...all the volumes make compulsive reading... they are, primarily, important historical records'.
British Medical Journal (2002) **325:** 1119, review of the series

Technology transfer in Britain: The case of monoclonal antibodies
Self and non-self: A history of autoimmunity
Endogenous opiates
The Committee on Safety of Drugs
In: Tansey E M, Catterall P P, Christie D A, Willhoft S V, Reynolds L A. (eds) (1997) *Wellcome Witnesses to Twentieth Century Medicine*. Volume 1. London: The Wellcome Trust, 135pp. ISBN 1 869835 79 4

Making the human body transparent: The impact of NMR and MRI
Research in general practice
Drugs in psychiatric practice
The MRC Common Cold Unit
In: Tansey E M, Christie D A, Reynolds L A. (eds) (1998) *Wellcome Witnesses to Twentieth Century Medicine*. Volume 2. London: The Wellcome Trust, 282pp. ISBN 1 869835 39 5

Early heart transplant surgery in the UK
In: Tansey E M, Reynolds L A. (eds) (1999) *Wellcome Witnesses to Twentieth Century Medicine*. Volume 3. London: The Wellcome Trust, 72pp. ISBN 1 841290 07 6

Haemophilia: Recent history of clinical management
In: Tansey E M, Christie D A. (eds) (1999) *Wellcome Witnesses to Twentieth Century Medicine*. Volume 4. London: The Wellcome Trust, 90pp. ISBN 1 841290 08 4

Looking at the unborn: Historical aspects of obstetric ultrasound
In: Tansey E M, Christie D A. (eds) (2000) *Wellcome Witnesses to Twentieth Century Medicine*. Volume 5. London: The Wellcome Trust, 80pp. ISBN 1 841290 11 4

Post penicillin antibiotics: From acceptance to resistance?
In: Tansey E M, Reynolds L A. (eds) (2000) *Wellcome Witnesses to Twentieth Century Medicine*. Volume 6. London: The Wellcome Trust, 71pp.
ISBN 1 841290 12 2

Clinical research in Britain, 1950–1980
In: Reynolds L A, Tansey E M. (eds) (2000) *Wellcome Witnesses to Twentieth Century Medicine*. Volume 7. London: The Wellcome Trust, 74pp.
ISBN 1 841290 16 5

Intestinal absorption
In: Christie D A, Tansey E M. (eds) (2000) *Wellcome Witnesses to Twentieth Century Medicine*. Volume 8. London: The Wellcome Trust, 81pp.
ISBN 1 841290 17 3

Neonatal intensive care
In: Christie D A, Tansey E M. (eds) (2001) *Wellcome Witnesses to Twentieth Century Medicine*. Volume 9. London: The Wellcome Trust Centre for the History of Medicine at UCL, 84pp. ISBN 0 854840 76 1

British contributions to medical research and education in Africa after the Second World War
In: Reynolds L A, Tansey E M. (eds) (2001) *Wellcome Witnesses to Twentieth Century Medicine*. Volume 10. London: The Wellcome Trust Centre for the History of Medicine at UCL, 93pp. ISBN 0 854840 77 X

Childhood asthma and beyond
In: Reynolds L A, Tansey E M. (eds) (2001) *Wellcome Witnesses to Twentieth Century Medicine*. Volume 11. London: The Wellcome Trust Centre for the History of Medicine at UCL, 74pp. ISBN 0 854840 78 8

Maternal care
In: Christie D A, Tansey E M. (eds) (2001) *Wellcome Witnesses to Twentieth Century Medicine*. Volume 12. London: The Wellcome Trust Centre for the History of Medicine at UCL, 88pp. ISBN 0 854840 79 6

Population-based research in south Wales: The MRC Pneumoconiosis Research Unit and the MRC Epidemiology Unit
In: Ness A R, Reynolds L A, Tansey E M. (eds) (2002) *Wellcome Witnesses to Twentieth Century Medicine*. Volume 13. London: The Wellcome Trust Centre for the History of Medicine at UCL, 74pp. ISBN 0 854840 81 8

Peptic ulcer: Rise and fall
In: Christie D A, Tansey E M. (eds) (2002) *Wellcome Witnesses to Twentieth Century Medicine*. Volume 14. London: The Wellcome Trust Centre for the History of Medicine at UCL, 143pp. ISBN 0 854840 84 2

Leukaemia
In: Christie D A, Tansey E M. (eds) (2003) *Wellcome Witnesses to Twentieth Century Medicine*. Volume 15. London: The Wellcome Trust Centre for the History of Medicine at UCL, 86pp. ISBN 0 85484 087 7

The MRC Applied Psychology Unit
In: Reynolds L A, Tansey E M. (eds) (2003) *Wellcome Witnesses to Twentieth Century Medicine*. Volume 16. London: The Wellcome Trust Centre for the History of Medicine at UCL, 94pp. ISBN 0 85484 088 5

Genetic testing
In: Christie D A, Tansey E M. (eds) (2003) *Wellcome Witnesses to Twentieth Century Medicine*. Volume 17. London: The Wellcome Trust Centre for the History of Medicine at UCL, 130pp. ISBN 0 85484 094 X

Foot and mouth disease: The 1967 outbreak and its aftermath
In: Reynolds L A, Tansey E M. (eds) (2003) *Wellcome Witnesses to Twentieth Century Medicine*. Volume 18. London: The Wellcome Trust Centre for the History of Medicine at UCL, 114pp. ISBN 0 85484 096 6

Environmental toxicology: The legacy of *Silent Spring*
In: Christie D A, Tansey E M. (eds) (2004) *Wellcome Witnesses to Twentieth Century Medicine*. Volume 19. London: The Wellcome Trust Centre for the History of Medicine at UCL, 132pp. ISBN 0 85484 091 5

Cystic fibrosis
In: Christie D A, Tansey E M. (eds) (2004) *Wellcome Witnesses to Twentieth Century Medicine*. Volume 20. London: The Wellcome Trust Centre for the History of Medicine at UCL, 120pp. ISBN 0 85484 086 9

Innovation in pain management
In: Reynolds L A, Tansey E M. (eds) (2004) *Wellcome Witnesses to Twentieth Century Medicine*. Volume 21. London: The Wellcome Trust Centre for the History of Medicine at UCL, 125pp. ISBN 0 85484 097 4

The Rhesus factor and disease prevention
In: Zallen D T, Christie D A, Tansey E M. (eds) (2004) *Wellcome Witnesses to Twentieth Century Medicine*. Volume 22. London: The Wellcome Trust Centre for the History of Medicine at UCL, 98pp. ISBN 0 85484 099 0

The recent history of platelets in thrombosis and other disorders
In: Reynolds L A, Tansey E M. (eds) (2005) *Wellcome Witnesses to Twentieth Century Medicine*. Volume 23. London: The Wellcome Trust Centre for the History of Medicine at UCL, 186pp. ISBN 0 85484 103 2

Short-course chemotherapy for tuberculosis
In: Christie D A, Tansey E M. (eds) (2005) *Wellcome Witnesses to Twentieth Century Medicine*. Volume 24. London: The Wellcome Trust Centre for the History of Medicine at UCL, 120pp. ISBN 0 85484 104 0

Prenatal corticosteroids for reducing morbidity and mortality after preterm birth
In: Reynolds L A, Tansey E M. (eds) (2005) *Wellcome Witnesses to Twentieth Century Medicine*. Volume 25. London: The Wellcome Trust Centre for the History of Medicine at UCL, 154pp. ISBN 0 85484 102 4

Public health in the 1980s and 1990s: Decline and rise?
In: Berridge V, Christie D A, Tansey E M. (eds) (2006) *Wellcome Witnesses to Twentieth Century Medicine*. Volume 26. London: The Wellcome Trust Centre for the History of Medicine at UCL, 101pp. ISBN 0 85484 106 7

Cholesterol, atherosclerosis and coronary disease in the UK, 1950–2000
In: Reynolds L A, Tansey E M. (eds) (2006) *Wellcome Witnesses to Twentieth Century Medicine*. Volume 27. London: The Wellcome Trust Centre for the History of Medicine at UCL. This volume. ISBN 0 85484 107 5.

The development of physics applied to medicine in the UK, 1945–90
In: Christie D A, Tansey E M. (eds) (2006) *Wellcome Witnesses to Twentieth Century Medicine*. Volume 28. The Wellcome Trust Centre for the History of Medicine at UCL. In press.

Volumes 1–12 cost £5 plus postage, with volumes 13–20 at £10 each. Orders of four or more volumes receive a 20 per cent discount. All 20 published volumes in the series are available at the special price of £115 plus postage. To order a copy contact t.tillotson@wellcome.ac.uk or by phone: +44 (0)207 611 8486; or fax: +44 (0)207 611 8703.

All volumes are freely available online at www.ucl.ac.uk/histmed following the links to Publications/Wellcome Witnesses.

Copies of volumes 21–27 can be ordered from www.amazon.co.uk; www.amazon.com; and all good booksellers for £6/$10 plus postage.

Other publications

Technology transfer in Britain: The case of monoclonal antibodies
In: Tansey E M, Catterall P P. (1993) *Contemporary Record* **9:** 409–44.

Monoclonal antibodies: A witness seminar on contemporary medical history
In: Tansey E M, Catterall P P. (1994) *Medical History* **38:** 322–7.

Chronic pulmonary disease in South Wales coalmines: An eye-witness account of the MRC surveys (1937–42)
In: P D'Arcy Hart, edited and annotated by E M Tansey. (1998) *Social History of Medicine* **11:** 459–68.

Ashes to Ashes – The history of smoking and health
In: Lock S P, Reynolds L A, Tansey E M. (eds) (1998) Amsterdam: Rodopi BV, 228pp. ISBN 90420 0396 0 (Hfl 125) (hardback). Reprinted 2003.

Witnessing medical history. An interview with Dr Rosemary Biggs
Professor Christine Lee and Dr Charles Rizza (interviewers). (1998) *Haemophilia* **4:** 769–77.

Witnessing the Witnesses: Pitfalls and potentials of the Witness Seminar in twentieth century medicine
By E M Tansey. In: Doel R, Soderqvist T. (eds) (2006) *Writing Recent Science: The historiography of contemporary science, technology and medicine***.** London: Routledge.

INTRODUCTION

Plasma cholesterol as a cause of coronary heart disease (CHD); the cholesterol–CHD hypothesis

During the years following the Second World War, the standardized death rate from coronary heart disease (CHD) in men increased sharply in Western industrialized countries. When the search for the causes of this increase in CHD began, plasma cholesterol was already a prime suspect. It had long been known that cholesterol is a major component of advanced atherosclerotic lesions in humans and that atherosclerosis could be induced in animals by feeding cholesterol (see page 13). Another reason for fingering cholesterol was the recognition that hypercholesterolaemia due to a mutation in a single gene [the familial hypercholesterolaemia (FH) gene] is strongly associated with CHD (see pages 29–30). It was hard to argue that in this case CHD was not caused by the hypercholesterolaemia.

Case-control studies in the early 1950s showed that in patients with CHD the plasma low-density lipoprotein (LDL) cholesterol level was higher than in normal controls.[2] In the US Framingham prospective study of over 5000 healthy men and women followed for more than 30 years, the risk of developing CHD was proportional to the plasma total and LDL cholesterol level at entry into the study.[3] The results of this and other prospective studies were used in the design of large-scale clinical trials to test the effect of reducing the plasma cholesterol level on CHD incidence. Early trials were disappointing,[4] probably because the fall in plasma cholesterol levels achieved in the treated groups was too small to provide sufficient statistical power. The most successful of the 'pre-statin' trials was the 1984 US Lipid Research Clinics' Coronary Primary Prevention Trial (see Table 2, page 76).[5] In the treated group the mean fall in plasma cholesterol was small, but there was a statistically significant decrease in CHD events. Reactions to this result were mixed. Some among the US medical community considered that the trial warranted a national campaign to lower cholesterol

---

[2] Barr *et al.* (1951).

[3] Gordon *et al.* (1977).

[4] Frantz and Moore (1969).

[5] Lipid Research Clinics (LRC) Coronary Primary Prevention Trial (1984): 351–64.

levels in the US population. Others began a campaign to discredit its organizers. This ill-tempered controversy continued for many years on both sides of the Atlantic, prompting one of the organizers of the trial to recount the history of this controversy in a forthcoming book entitled *The Cholesterol Wars.*[6]

When statins became available for clinical use (see below), several trials with a much better prospect of achieving statistical significance were carried out in Scandinavia, Scotland, the US and Australia.[7] The results of these trials, reported between 1994 and 1998, showed beyond doubt that a reduction in plasma cholesterol level significantly reduces CHD incidence in selected populations. These results have now been extended by a trial in which Sir Richard Doll (1912–2005), one of the architects of the modern clinical trial, played a leading role.[8] In this trial, involving more than 20 000 UK adults, simvastatin significantly reduced the CHD event rate in men and women, including those whose LDL cholesterol levels were near the lower limit of the normal range.

The 30 or more steps in the biosynthesis of cholesterol from acetyl-CoA were elucidated by several groups, roughly between the early 1950s and the mid-1970s. The main players were John Cornforth and George Popják (my boss at Hammersmith from 1954–62) in Britain; Konrad Bloch and Robert Burns Woodward at Harvard; and Feodor Lynen in Munich. Four of the five were awarded the Nobel Prize for this work.[9] In the opinion of many, Popják should have shared the prize, but this was not to be. A key event in the story was the finding that an essential step in cholesterol synthesis is the formation of units of a branched-chain C_5 compound (isoprenoid units) that give rise to the carbon skeleton of cholesterol.[10] The breakthrough in the search for the isoprenoid unit

---

[6] Four extensive excerpts from the forthcoming book by Professor Daniel Steinberg have been published to date in the *Journal of Lipid Research* [Steinberg (2004, 2005a and b, 2006)]. The 1984 trial is discussed in Steinberg (2006).

[7] Scandinavian Simvastatin Survival Study (4S) (1994); Shepherd *et al.* for the West of Scotland Coronary Prevention Study Group (1995); Sacks *et al.* for the Cholesterol and Recurrent Events Trial Investigators (1996) ; The Long-term Intervention with Pravastatin in Ischemic Disease (LIPID) Study Group (1998).

[8] Heart Protection Study Collaborative Group (2002).

[9] Konrad Bloch and Feodor Lynen shared the Nobel Prize in Physiology or Medicine for 1964 for their discoveries concerning the mechanism and regulation of the cholesterol and fatty acid metabolism; and Robert Burns Woodward received the Nobel Prize in Chemistry in 1965 for his outstanding achievements in the art of organic synthesis; and John Cornforth shared the Nobel Prize in Chemistry for 1975 for his work on the stereochemistry of enzyme-catalyzed reactions.

[10] Cornforth (1959).

was the serendipitous discovery of a C_6 acid (mevalonic acid or MVA) by a group of microbiologists searching for growth factors for *Lactobacillus acidophilus.*[11] When MVA turned out to be an extremely efficient precursor for cholesterol synthesis *in vitro*, they suggested, correctly, that MVA is decarboxylated to give the C_5 isoprenoid. There followed the discovery by several independent groups that MVA is formed in yeast and animal cells by the reduction of 3-hydroxy-3-methylglutaryl coenzyme A (HMG-CoA) by the enzyme HMG-CoA reductase.[12]

In 1957 Gordon Gould, a charming American who was learning to play the bassoon, joined Popják's lab for a year's sabbatical. He spent his first few months writing a couple of chapters for Cook's book, to the mild annoyance of Popják.[13] But he more than made up for this by showing, with Popják, that when the incorporation of ^{14}C-acetate into the cholesterol of a rat's liver is inhibited by feeding cholesterol, there is no change in the rate of incorporation of ^{14}C-MVA.[14] This showed that the rate-limiting step in cholesterol biosynthesis lies before MVA. Marvin Siperstein and Violet Fagan then showed that the reduction of HMG-CoA to MVA by HMG-CoA reductase is the step that determines the rate of synthesis of cholesterol in the liver.[15]

Popják was medically qualified and had begun his career as a pathologist with an interest in atherosclerosis. When I joined his MRC unit at Hammersmith he was a card-carrying believer in the cholesterol–CHD hypothesis, but he had turned himself into a lipid biochemist hoping, so he told me, that an understanding of cholesterol biosynthesis would contribute to the treatment of CHD. The feasibility of inhibiting one of the steps in cholesterol synthesis in a clinical setting was discussed in Popják's lab, but as far as I know Popják never explored the possibility of inhibiting HMG-CoA reductase. Had Popják thought of asking Cornforth to synthesize an analogue of HMG-CoA, they might have discovered the first inhibitor of HMG-CoA reductase. In fact, the specific inhibition of this enzyme was first achieved by a group of Japanese microbiologists.[16]

---

[11] Wright *et al.* (1956).

[12] Cornforth (1973).

[13] Cook (ed.) (1958).

[14] Gould and Popják (1957).

[15] Siperstein and Fagan (1964).

[16] Endo *et al.* (1976b).

When Barry Lewis joined my MRC group in 1963 to collaborate in the investigation of hyperlipidaemia, we set up a Lipid Clinic at Hammersmith. This was the first such clinic in Britain. Our first patient was a 10-year-old Iraqi girl with extensive skin xanthomas present since age 4 and a plasma cholesterol level of 800–900mg/100ml. Both her parents were hypercholesterolaemic and her brother and sister had died from CHD aged 15 and 9. The patient's plasma cholesterol level showed little or no response to corn oil, cholestyramine, *Atromid,* D-thyroxine or neomycin. We therefore decided to try the effect of plasmapheresis. In September 1964, on each of four consecutive days, 500ml of blood were taken from the patient. The blood was centrifuged and the red cells immediately transfused into her. This procedure resulted in a fall in plasma cholesterol from 830mg/100ml to 525mg/100ml, but the level returned to the baseline value within a few weeks. We did not repeat the procedure. The patient died at age 13, after repeated attacks of angina at rest. A post mortem was not done. To add to the misfortunes of this family the patient's father, who became the Prime Minister of Iraq, was imprisoned and hanged after the Ba'th coup of 1968.

As a member of Popják's MRC unit at Hammersmith Hospital, I built up a small team whose aim was to combine biochemical with clinical lipidology. In 1962 the MRC and the Postgraduate School agreed to my taking on a clinical collaborator and to our having the use of four hospital beds. This was the agreement under which Barry Lewis joined me (1963–65). By 1969 our group had grown to 11 people. When William Hayes' MRC Microbial Genetics Unit moved from Hammersmith Hospital to Edinburgh I asked the MRC to convert my team into a Unit accommodated in the space in the Cyclotron Building left by Hayes. This was agreed and in 1969 we became the MRC Lipid Metabolism Unit. Our brief included 'investigation and treatment of patients with disorders of plasma lipid metabolism, particularly those leading to ischaemic heart disease'. The Unit was closed on my retirement in 1983.

In 1976 a group headed by Endo, working in a laboratory of the Sankyo drug company, isolated a compound (compactin, see page 79) from *Penicillium citrinum.*[17] They noted that a portion of the compactin molecule bore a striking stereochemical resemblance to HMG-CoA. They then showed that compactin is a powerful inhibitor of HMG-CoA reductase, and that when given to dogs it lowered the plasma cholesterol level. Within a few years of its discovery,

[17] Endo *et al.* (1976b).

compactin was shown to lower total and LDL cholesterol levels in heterozygous FH patients, without significant clinical or biochemical side-effects.

Compactin itself never became generally available for clinical use, but in 1980 Merck Research Laboratories reported the isolation of a more potent inhibitor of HMG-CoA reductase from the fungus *Aspergillus terreus.*[18] This compound, called lovastatin, was shown to lower the plasma LDL cholesterol level by at least 50 per cent in normal humans and FH heterozygotes without side-effects when given at a maximum dose rate of 80mg/day (see page 36). Lovastatin is now available for prescription use in the US, but not in the UK. Several other inhibitory analogues of compactin have now been described and are known as statins. The safety and effectiveness of statins opened the way for the definitive clinical trials discussed above, and raised the possibility of primary prevention of CHD in well populations.[19]

Nick Myant
Hammersmith Hospital

[18] Alberts *et al.* (1980). See also Vagelos and Galambos (2004): 132–63.

[19] Durrington (2004).

CHOLESTEROL, ATHEROSCLEROSIS AND CORONARY DISEASE IN THE UK, 1950–2000

The transcript of a Witness Seminar held by the Wellcome Trust Centre for the History of Medicine at UCL, London, on 8 March 2005

Edited by L A Reynolds and E M Tansey

CHOLESTEROL, ATHEROSCLEROSIS AND CORONARY DISEASE IN THE UK, 1950–2000

Participants

Professor David Barker
Professor John Betteridge
Sir Christopher Booth
Professor Gustav Born
Professor Richard Bruckdorfer
Professor George Davey Smith
Professor Paul Durrington
Professor David Galton
Dr Arthur Hollman
Professor Steve Humphries
Professor Gordon Lowe
Professor Vincent Marks
Dr Paul Miller
Professor Jerry Morris
Professor Michael Oliver (Chair)
Professor Chris Packard
Professor Stuart Pocock
Professor Kalevi Pyörälä
Professor Thomas Sanders
Professor James Scott
Dr Elspeth Smith
Professor Anne Soutar
Professor Gilbert Thompson
Professor Hugh Tunstall-Pedoe
Professor Neville Woolf
Professor John S Yudkin

Among those attending the meeting: Mr Owen Davies, Mr Miguel Garcia-Sancho, Professor Jeremy Pearson, Professor Sir Stanley Peart, Dr Tim Powell, Professor Hilary Rose, Dr Ronald Smith, Mr John Stewart

Apologies include: Professor Dame Carol Black, Dr David Bowyer, Dr Michael Burr, Professor Rory Collins, Dr Huw Dorkins, Professor Christopher Edwards, Professor Peter Elwood, Professor Gerald Fowkes, Dr Joseph Goldstein, Professor Austin Gresham, Professor Walter Holland, Professor Malcolm Law, Dr Barry Lewis, Professor Ross Lorimer, Professor Sir Michael Marmot, Dr Norman Miller, Dr Malcolm Mitchinson, Dr Nick Myant, Professor Lawrence Ramsay, Professor Gerry Shaper, Professor James Shepherd, Dr Joan Slack, Professor Nicholas Wald, Professor Kenneth Walton, Professor Peter Weissberg

Sir Christopher Booth: Ladies and gentlemen, may I warmly welcome you today. I am standing in for Tilli Tansey, Convenor of the History of Twentieth Century Medicine Group, who would have been here today, but sadly, she has a bad attack of the flu and sends her apologies.

A Witness Seminar brings together people who have actually been involved in a particular historical episode, to talk about the events in their working lives; to remember; to discuss and debate. As far as medicine is concerned, we found that the technique of a one-to-one interview on videotape was easily flawed, because it depended on the accuracy of the interviewer and how well he or she knew the science of the person being interviewed. We believe we get more truthful history from a Witness Seminar than we would from single interviews.

The Group have held more than 40 meetings, some of which are very useful historical documents. For example, the meeting on monoclonal antibodies included contributions from Dr Georges Köhler and Dr César Milstein.[1] That document is now of great historic significance, since they are both dead.

As, of course, this meeting will be a historic document, I hope, for some time in the future. I will hand over to Michael Oliver, who has kindly agreed to chair this meeting.

Professor Michael Oliver: It's very good to see so many familiar faces. Welcome to you all. As you realize, we are forcing you back 50 years or so ago to record what you were actually thinking about then, where and why. Elspeth Smith said to me in a letter, 'How can you possibly expect us to recall what we were thinking about half a century ago, when I can't remember what I was thinking about yesterday?'

The purpose of this meeting is to record what we, in the UK, were thinking about cholesterol and associated lipids, and their relation to cardiovascular, particularly coronary heart disease (CHD), in the last half of the twentieth century.

In the beginning of the 1940s, CHD was regarded as an inevitable result of ageing. For example, in the monograph, *Vascular Sclerosis*, Eli Moschcowitz from Boston wrote: 'Arteriosclerosis [cannot] be prevented, no more than grey hair or facial wrinkles'.[2] In the UK, Ryle and Russell wrote in 1949: 'It seems at present

[1] Tansey and Catterall (eds) (1997): 1–34.

[2] Moschcowitz (1942): 143.

remotely unlikely that we shall discover a "cure" for general arteriosclerosis or coronary artery disease'.[3] Enthusiasm for research into its causes or therapy did not arise before the 1950s.

Appreciation of a possible causal link between raised blood cholesterol and heart disease had been suggested in the US by Paul Dudley White in the 3rd edition (1947) of his textbook *Heart Disease*:

> The cause of atheroma of the coronary arteries as well as that of arteriosclerosis in general is unknown… The occasional finding of a high blood cholesterol content in a fasting case of CHD, especially in the young patient under 40, is in favour of a disturbance of fat metabolism, at least as one factor.[4]

In the UK, there was no mention of cholesterol or lipids in William Evans' influential 1948 book, *Cardiology*.[5] Nor of atherosclerosis as a cause of CHD. Price's 1949 textbook on medicine does not mention cholesterol, except in the context of gallstones.[6] Xanthomata were simply a skin disease and atheroma was due to hypertension. So far as I know, the first mention in the UK of any relationship between cholesterol and arterial disease was in Paul Wood's first edition of *Diseases of the Heart and Circulation* in 1950.[7] He wrote:

> Lipoid substances accumulate in the intima of the large arteries in a patchy irregular fashion, sometimes encroaching on the lumen. The lipoid nature of the deposits, their relatively frequent association with diabetes and hypercholesterolaemia, suggest some relation to fat metabolism…[but] consideration should be given to the possibility that raised cholesterol might result *from* CHD.[8]

Meanwhile, in 1949, Jack Gofman, a physicist working in the Donner Laboratory in the Berkeley campus of the University of California using an analytical ultracentrifuge, recognized that the lipoproteins of human blood are divided into two groups – low density lipoproteins and high density lipoproteins –

---

[3] Ryle and Russell (1949): 389.

[4] White (1947): 479.

[5] Evans (1948).

[6] Price (1950).

[7] Wood (1950).

[8] Wood (1950): 372–4. Emphasis added by Professor Michael Oliver.

according to their densities (LDL: below 1.05g/ml; HDL: above 1.05g/ml) and flotation rates.[9] He labelled the group with 12–20 Svedberg flotation units [S_f], which we now know as LDL, to be 'atherosclerogenic'.[10]

This idea was not immediately taken up in the US and not at all in the UK. A month ago [February 2005] I spoke to Jack Gofman, now over 90 years of age, and he believes that his views were ignored largely because he was a physicist and not part of the orthodox medical scientific community. I can remember these analyses from the ultracentrifuge being dismissed as irrelevant and artificial in 1952, when I began working on the subject. Anyway, nobody in the UK had any money to buy an ultracentrifuge. It did not help when Ancel Keys, who submitted Gofman's data to detailed statistical analysis, claimed in 1951 that 'the use of lipoprotein classes as a discriminator between atherosclerosis and normal persons is no better than total cholesterol alone'.[11]

In the early 1950s, three other groups had begun to study lipoproteins: David Barr in New York used a low temperature chemical fractionation procedure that was laborious and required 25ml of serum;[12] Esko Nikkilä in Helsinki used filter-paper zone electrophoresis;[13] and in Edinburgh in 1953 George Boyd developed a filter-paper zone electrophoresis microtechnique using 0.1ml serum.[14] Our method was tedious, since it involved elution of cholesterol from 18 separate 1cm strips of Whatman paper and a run of eight hours. The latter was particularly tiresome, since there was no automated switch to stop the electrophoresis run, and George and I had to take it in turns to return to the lab between 11 pm and 12 midnight.

Ours was the first report in the UK in 1955 of the distribution of cholesterol between the α and β lipoproteins in men aged 50 years or under with CHD and age-matched controls.[15] We found 19 per cent more cholesterol on the β fraction and also an absolute decrease in the α fraction in men with CHD. The

---

[9] Gofman *et al.* (1949).

[10] Gofman *et al.* (1950, 1952) S_f = Svedberg flotation units, see Glossary, page 146.

[11] Keys (1951).

[12] Barr *et al.* (1951).

[13] Nikkilä (1953).

[14] Boyd (1954).

[15] Oliver and Boyd (1955).

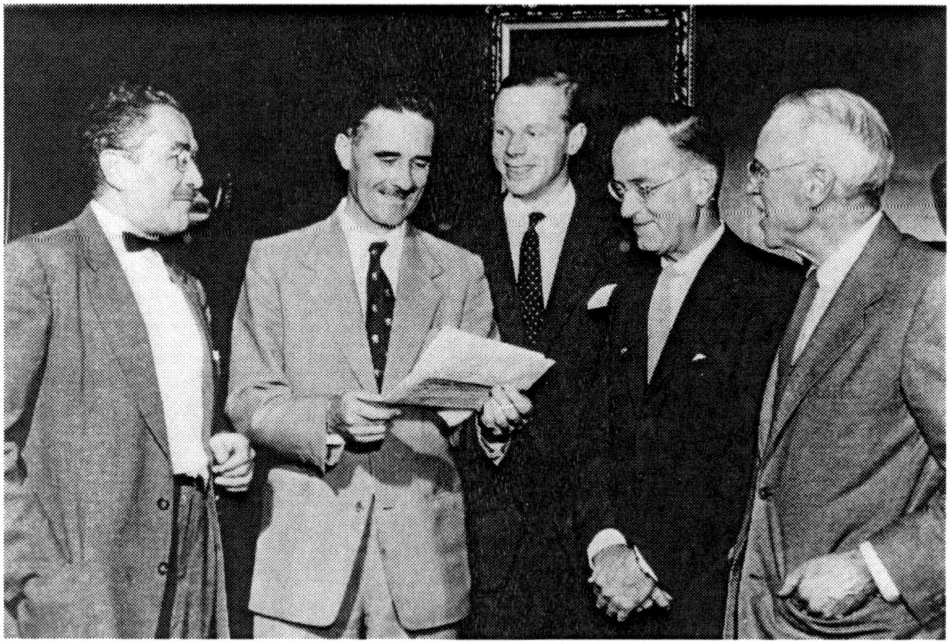

Figure 1: Ancel Keys' first international symposium on atherosclerosis in Minneapolis–St Paul, 1955. L to R: Louis Katz, Jack Brock, Michael Oliver, Irvine Page, Paul Dudley White.

β/α ratio was in the region of 10 in men with CHD and 2.6 in the controls. These are similar to the more familiar ratios of today regarding LDL/HDL in hypercholesterolaemic people and were reported at the First International Symposium on Atherosclerosis in 1955 [Figure 1].[16]

Previously, in 1953, we had reported a study of plasma lipids in 200 consecutive patients with CHD, and 200 age- and gender-matched controls.[17] This was the first UK study and at that time was the largest in the world.[18] There was significant elevation of plasma total cholesterol and the plasma total cholesterol/ phospholipid ratio in the coronary patients at all ages.

When I presented these results in a ten-minute paper at the 1953 Newcastle meeting of the British Cardiac Society, there was total silence.[19] No one asked

[16] Keys (ed.) (1955).

[17] Oliver and Boyd (1953c).

[18] For a discussion of the statistical obstacles accompanying large sample sizes, see Ness *et al.* (eds) (2002): 77–80.

[19] Oliver and Boyd (1953c).

any questions. Paul Wood said that this was 'irrelevant to cardiology' and that we should proceed to more important communications. Maurice Campbell, the President of the Society, commented, 'Let's not be too hasty, there might just be something in this cholesterol issue'.

The first paper on cholesterol that I published with George Boyd – who died from a coronary in 1983 aged only 59 – was earlier. In 1953 we studied changes in plasma cholesterol and total phospholipids during the menstrual cycle.[20] These were derived from daily blood samples taken from 12 young women over five weeks with early morning oral temperature measurements to identify ovulation. The results showed that the point of lowest plasma cholesterol occurred when oestrogen activity was maximal. We regarded this as possibly contributing to the rarity of CHD in premenopausal women. This study led us into five years of intensive research into the effects of various hormones and endocrine states on plasma lipids and lipoproteins.[21]

At about this time, 1956, John Cornforth at the National Institute for Medical Research at Mill Hill, London, and George Popják at the Hammersmith Hospital, London, were studying the biosynthesis of cholesterol from acetate.[22] They speculated about the possibility of inhibiting key enzymes to reduce the synthesis of 3-hydroxy-3-methylglutarate-CoA (HMG-CoA). It took more than 20 years before their proposals reached fruition, leading to the development of the first statins in the 1980s.[23] In 1958, Cook in Dundee published a book on the physiology and biochemistry of cholesterol.[24]

Now I shall ask Gilbert Thompson to describe the development of interest in cholesterol and lipoproteins in the 1960s and onwards – and [Sir John] McMichael's influential dismissal of the whole idea.

Professor Gilbert Thompson: Thank you very much, Michael, for inviting me here to say something about my early knowledge of lipidology, which is not as lengthy as yours. I was still a medical student when you and Boyd were

---

[20] Oliver and Boyd (1953a).

[21] Boyd and Oliver (1956).

[22] Cornforth *et al.* (1954); Popják (1958). Mill Hill is the location of the Medical Research Council's National Institute for Medical Research in north London.

[23] Endo *et al.* (1977).

[24] Cook (ed.) (1958).

producing the results of your early research. My memories start in 1965 when I was working with Chris Booth and we were interested in looking at vitamin D metabolism in patients with malabsorption. We set up an absorption test, and got hold of some vitamin D to radiolabel. Thanks to advice from Barry Lewis, I managed to tritiate the vitamin D rather than everything else in the lab and our absorption test went quite well.[25] The following year I went to the Massachusetts General Hospital in Boston to continue my research. In 1967 Fredrickson, Levy and Lees produced their five-part paper in the *New England Journal of Medicine*.[26] Suddenly everybody in Boston seemed to be thinking and talking about cholesterol and lipoproteins, including a couple of very bright interns at the Massachusetts General Hospital called Goldstein and Brown.[27]

I went back to the Hammersmith, where Chris Booth was by now Professor of Medicine, because Sir John McMichael had retired, and I continued to do some research on vitamin D, although I was getting increasingly interested in atherosclerosis and cholesterol. A couple of years later I went to see Graham Bull at Northwick Park, to see whether there was any opening for that line of research, but he thought it was not a very promising one. In 1972 I managed to persuade Chris Booth to give me a year's leave of absence and I went to work with Tony Gotto in Houston, where I first met Anne Soutar, and got increasingly involved with apolipoproteins and their metabolism. I came back again to the Hammersmith, still trying to do gastroenterology, although I was really more interested in lipidology, which, of course, didn't exist as a specialty in those days.

In 1974 John Yudkin's uncle, a namesake I think, who was Emeritus Professor of Nutrition at Queen Elizabeth College, London, wrote an article in *The Times* about the role of sugar in coronary disease.[28] I persuaded *The Times* to let me rebut this in an article.[29] This led to a BBC debate that was televised at the Royal Institution. Don Fredrickson, Peter Taggart and I were up against Yudkin

---

[25] Thompson *et al.* (1966).

[26] Fredrickson *et al.* (1967).

[27] Goldstein and Brown (1977). Michael Brown and Joseph Goldstein shared the Nobel Prize for Physiology or Medicine in 1985 for their discoveries concerning the regulation of cholesterol metabolism. See their biographical notes on pages 125 and 127.

[28] Yudkin J (1974).

[29] Thompson (1974).

and it created a certain amount of interest.[30] One thing led to another, and eventually in 1975 I gave up gastroenterology, joined Nick Myant's Medical Research Council (MRC)'s Lipid Metabolism Unit,[31] which had been created about five years previously and helped him organize a memorable meeting at the Hammersmith [see Figure 2]. As most of you know, Nick is probably the founding father of lipid research in this country and a man of enormous intellect, but great modesty, and many of us owe him a lot.[32] He had been McMichael's houseman, which was a bit ironic, seeing as their views differed diametrically.

Before I finish I would like to mention one other debate, which took place in Rotterdam in 1977 under the aegis of the European Society of Clinical Investigation, the motion being 'that modification of serum lipids by dietary and/or other means will influence the incidence of, or mortality from, coronary heart disease'.[33] Shlomo Eisenberg, Lars Carlson and I supported the motion, with McMichael, Paul Astrup and Christian Crone against. Crone showed two slides: one of a lovely, glossy-coated rat, which he said had been brought up on butter; and the other was a miserable, mangey-looking specimen which he said had been brought up on polyunsaturated fat. The audience dissolved into laughter and that was the end of the debate. Sir John McMichael was jubilant about this, not surprisingly, for although he had retired, he was by no means inactive. He was sending streams of letters to the *Lancet* and his cup was filled to overflowing when Michael Oliver published the results of the WHO trial, which showed that although nonfatal myocardial infarcts (MIs) were reduced by clofibrate, deaths from noncardiovascular causes increased.[34]

---

[30] The debate, held on 4 September 1974 with Professor Sir George Porter in the chair, was broadcast by BBC2 on 30 September 1974 as 'Controversy: The dietary cause of heart disease is sugar not fat' and the producer was Dominic Flessati. Neither the BBC nor the National Film and Television Archive hold a copy of this programme in their collections and *The Listener* did not publish a summary. We are grateful to Professor Thompson for a copy of the announcement of the debate, which will be deposited along with the tapes and other records of the meeting in Archives and Manuscripts, Wellcome Library, London.

[31] The MRC Lipid Metabolism Unit at Hammersmith Hospital, London, was established in 1969 to study lipid metabolism, particularly in relation to the problem of atherosclerosis, and was directed by Dr Nick Myant until it was disbanded on his retirement in 1983. See Thomson (1975, 1987): 368. See also Introduction.

[32] Myant (1990a and b).

[33] The European Society for Clinical Investigation's 'Controversy in Medicine' debate was held at the annual meeting in Rotterdam on 21 April 1977, chaired by Dr R Hermon Dowling.

[34] Principal Investigators (1978, 1984).

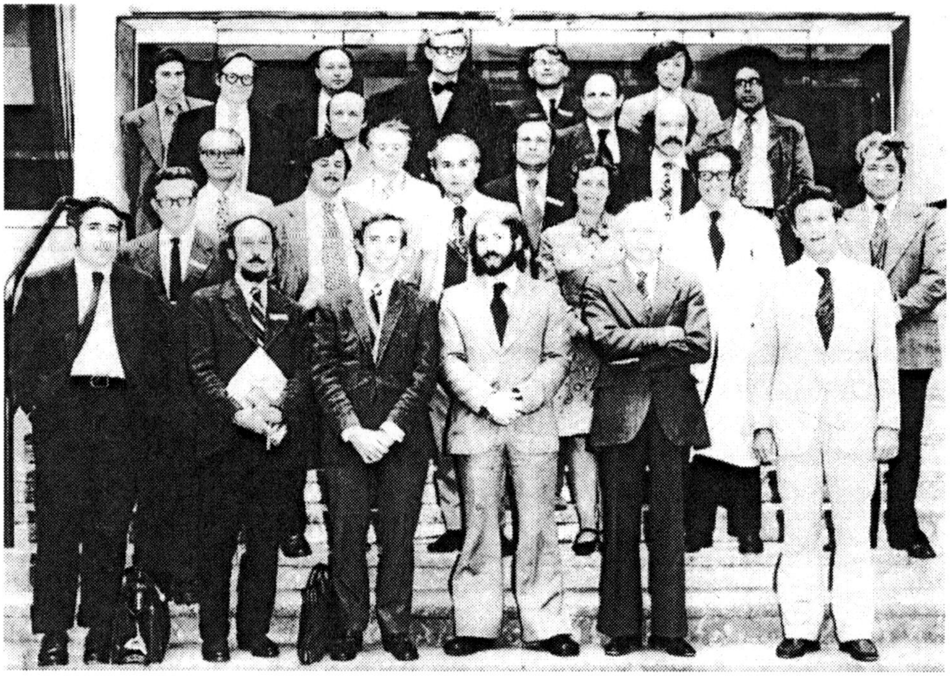

Figure 2: Participants at the Workshop on Familial Hypercholesterolaemia held at the Hammersmith Hospital, London, in 1975.

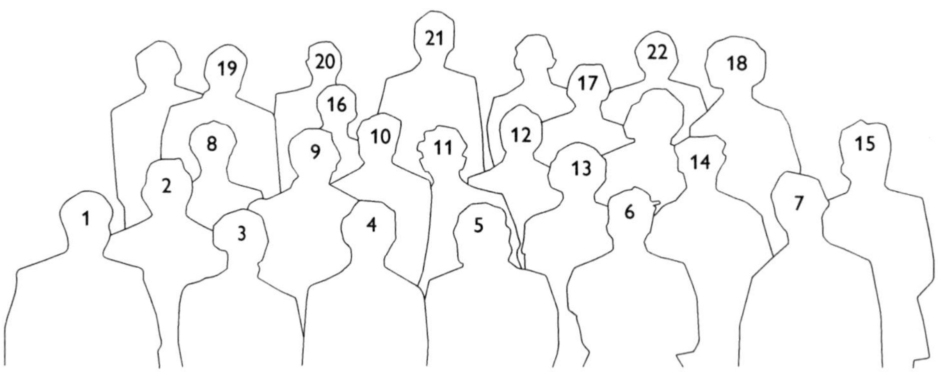

Key. L to R: 1: R Levy; 2: R Lees; 3: D Steinberg; 4: A Gotto; 5: M Press; 6: N Myant; 7: G Thompson; 8: A Kharchadurian; 9: M Brown; 10: J Goldstein; 11: G Popják; 12: D Bilheimer; 13: J Slack; 14: B Lewis; 15: K Mitropoulos; 16: T Miettinen; 17: D Reichl; 18: H Magnani; 19: S Grundy; 20: J de Gennes; 21: K Hellstrom; 22: G Gibbons.
From Thompson (1999): 32.

Sir John McMichael came out in the *British Medical Journal* (*BMJ*) with an article entitled 'Fats and atheroma: an inquest', and as far as he was concerned that was the end of it.[35] He was a great man, I have enormous respect for him, but he had a complete blind spot about cholesterol. I am afraid he was totally wrong about this, but because of his reputation and influence, he completely altered the whole climate of cardiology, certainly among senior cardiologists. To illustrate this point I want to read a very brief excerpt from a letter that I received from a general practitioner:

> Mr Edwards is a 38-year-old man who underwent an extensive coronary artery bypass operation in December 1987; his post-operative recovery was physically uneventful. However, we were quite concerned about our inability to reduce his high cholesterol and triglyceride levels. That was in August 1988. His cholesterol was 8.4 to 9.5 and triglyceride 3.3 to 5.3. Mr Edwards was getting very screwed up about his inability to drop his cholesterol and triglyceride and was very frightened that his new coronary arteries were soon to get furred up. As a result of this I referred him to the Brompton Hospital. He saw a consultant cardiologist, who told him to forget taking any tablets, to forget his cholesterol and triglyceride and to go away and try and live a normal life. That advice caused us some considerable concern, as we had been working very hard for the last couple of years to reduce his cholesterol. He is now on no medication.

I rest my case.

Professor Chris Packard: I will pick up the story from where you left off. I did my apprenticeship in lipidology in the early 1970s, a period that coincided with the pioneering work of the MRC Lipid Metabolism Unit. Our basic approach was to isolate the lipoprotein particles themselves, label them in some way and then re-introduce them and follow the metabolic pathway. Gilbert has already alluded to the work of Shlomo Eisenberg, a key worker in this field.[36] He was the first person to label very low-density lipoprotein (VLDL) and show that the radioactivity ended up in LDL. That was the beginning of studies of the delipidation pathway. Terry Langer and Bob Levy, working in the National Institutes of Health (NIH), had performed many of the earlier studies looking at the metabolic defects in people with high cholesterol levels.

---

[35] McMichael (1979).

[36] Eisenberg *et al.* (1973); Anonymous (1996).

They demonstrated a delayed clearance, while people with low cholesterol levels could turn over LDL much faster.[37] In the 1970s Anne Soutar, Gil Thompson and ourselves at Glasgow began to describe the metabolic defects in familial hypercholesterolaemia.[38] Many other labs using similar techniques documented what happened in people with different forms of hypercholesterolaemia. Shortly after that, interestingly, the nomenclature that had been introduced by Professor Don Fredrickson[39] – type I, type II, type III, type IV, type V – was simplified greatly into raised cholesterol, raised triglyceride and combined hyperlipidaemia.[40] This was a benefit, in that common defects gave rise to elevations in VLDL and LDL. This work, combined with that of Tony Gotto and others who investigated the structure of lipoproteins, changed our picture of these little oil droplets floating around in the blood.[41] We began to understand that cholesterol was the cargo, and the protein around the surface of the particle was directing its metabolic fate. I think this was a paradigm set that took us into the early 1980s, when we began to move into the cell biology arena.

Professor Anne Soutar: It's a pleasure to be here and to see so many familiar faces. I must say it is just like the good old days when Elspeth Smith and I were the only women to be seen around. It takes me back to the days of our Atherosclerosis Discussion Group.[42]

I can't add very much because I also came out of the Tony Gotto stable and I went there not as a clinician, of course, but as a biochemist and enzymologist. When

---

[37] Levy and Langer (1971); Langer *et al.* (1972).

[38] Soutar *et al.* (1977); Shepherd *et al.* (1979).

[39] Fredrickson and Lees (1966). Chapter 22 on familial hyperlipoproteinaemia, pages 429–88, describes five types of essential hyperlipoproteinaemia, including type V for the first time. For greater detail of his thinking, see Fredrickson's annotations on his list of publications at http://profiles.nlm.nih.gov/FF/B/B/L/G/_/ffbblg.txt (visited 15 December 2005).

[40] Goldstein *et al.* (1973b).

[41] Smith *et al.* (1978).

[42] Professor Michael Oliver wrote: 'The Atherosclerosis Discussion Group was founded in 1961 by John French and Michael Oliver, with Lord Florey as the first Chairman. Meetings were held in the spring at Magdalen College, Oxford, and in the autumn at Jesus College, Cambridge. The emphasis was on an informal exchange of views on all aspects of atherosclerosis. The twice-yearly meetings continue and the discussion group is now called the British Atherosclerosis Society (BAS), the UK affiliate of the International Atherosclerosis Society (IAS).' Note on draft transcript, 25 November 2005. For further details see Reynolds and Tansey (eds) (2005): 26; and www.britathsoc.ac.uk/ (visited 12 December 2005).

I got there, they were interested in the enzymes that were involved in carrying out these complex metabolic processes that were clearly going on in the transfer of lipids, and they were trying to understand the structure of the lipoproteins. While I was there Richard Jackson and Jerry Segrest did their important work showing that the protein part of the lipoprotein formed an amphipathic alpha helix, with one side hydrophobic, interacting with lipid, and on the other side were hydrophilic residues that would interact with the water.[43] Suddenly it became possible to understand the structure of these particles and, of course, that was very important for the understanding of lipoprotein metabolism. As Chris [Packard] said, the proteins were the things that directed them around the body and allowed them to be taken up by the receptors. Those were very early days in Houston, when Brown and Goldstein identified the first LDL receptor, which I guess we will hear more of later.[44] It was a very exciting time to be in Texas. I had come from England to the US for the first time, to Houston, where you would see neon signs saying, '62 oz steak, free if you can eat it all'. In my opinion you could feed a family of six on that. But, on the other hand, if you went to the supermarkets, you couldn't buy butter, you couldn't buy cream, you couldn't buy cheese, because they had got the message, even by the early 1970s, that you weren't supposed to be eating saturated fat, and I think at that time they were trying to make a polyunsaturated cow, but I don't know whether that ever came about.[45] There was a particularly unattractive sort of cheese that you could buy, advertised as being 'fat-free'. Coming from a typical English diet, this seemed quite extraordinary and a huge contrast to what was going on in the UK at the time.

Professor David Galton: To go back to the early history: one of the objectives of this meeting is 'to identify our failings and errors', and one of them was that we completely ignored the German literature. In the early 1930s Thannhauser was classifying xanthomata and he was feeding cholesterol to dogs to induce atherosclerosis.[46] I came across his work, because he was exiled at the start of the Nazi period to Boston, and as I worked in his old lab there I got to know his work. Unfortunately I can't read German, so I don't know exactly what he found, but it was very much on the cholesterol–atheroma theme.

---

[43] Segrest *et al.* (1974).

[44] See note 77.

[45] Anonymous (1975a and b).

[46] Thannhauser (1940, 1950). See also note 49.

Oliver: Were xanthomata not regarded as simply a skin disease?

Galton: Yes, xanthomata were.

Oliver: Thinking that xanthomata might be part of a systemic disorder was not appreciated until the early 1950s.

Galton: No, in the German literature it was in the 1930s.

Dr Paul Miller: Carl Müller in the 1930s described what we would now call heterozygous familial hypercholesterolaemia (FH) as a cause of angina pectoris xanthomatosis and CHD.[47]

Oliver: In the British literature?

Miller: In the *Archives of Internal Medicine.* Gil will know.

Thompson: 1936.

Professor Kalevi Pyörälä: Professor Carl Müller from Oslo, Norway, carried out a very nice pedigree study of patients with FH and premature CHD, and published it in English in the late 1930s. This study sensitized the Norwegian medical community to cholesterol–CHD. There was another sensitization in Norway, namely the publication of a prospective epidemiological study on the relationship of serum cholesterol and CHD by Knut Westlund and Ragnar Nicolaysen.[48]

Booth: Could I just add that there has just been written a very good biographical note about Thannhauser by Alan Hofmann of California, and I think it's well worth getting hold of a copy.[49]

Professor Richard Bruckdorfer: Like Anne [Soutar], I was bought up as a biochemist, and during this period, the 1960s and 1970s, there was another parallel activity going on in relation to cholesterol, which was the role of cholesterol in cell membranes. There was enormous excitement about how it controlled membrane fluidity. Eventually these two paths, membrane cholesterol and lipoprotein cholesterol, did coalesce, but I think it was probably towards the end of the 1970s and the early 1980s before that happened. We didn't meet

[47] Müller (1939). Müller's study of 17 Oslo families began in 1936 and was published in 1939. Dr Paul Miller wrote: 'It is quite clear that Müller was describing FH as a cause of coronary disease and he published photographs of tendon xanthomata.' Letter to Mrs Lois Reynolds, 11 March 2006.

[48] Westlund and Nicolaysen (1966).

[49] Hofmann and Zöllner (2000).

at the same meetings, but we probably could have informed each other a lot better how this actually happened.

Professor Vincent Marks: I recall an interest in cholesterol from a clinical laboratory point of view. We in clinical biochemistry were really only interested in using cholesterol as a diagnostic test for thyroid disease, mainly myxoedema, and for liver and kidney disease. One of the advances came with the introduction first of paper, and then of cellulose acetate, electrophoresis for lipoproteins by Jim Kohn, later of Roehampton, but then at the Westminster Hospital Medical School.[50] With electrophoresis it was possible to separate the different lipoproteins, which previously had only been possible by centrifugation and this was not generally available. Cellulose acetate electrophoresis really brought us into the modern era and we started to distinguish between the different lipoprotein fractions. It was, however, a long time before their significance was generally appreciated. I was involved with a drug that was intended for use for lowering cholesterol.[51] It didn't lower cholesterol, but it did raise plasma α-lipoprotein [also known as α-lipoprotein, high-density lipoprotein or HDL] levels. This was not considered as relevant by the regulatory authorities at the time.

Oliver: We are into pathology now. Sadly, several of the pioneers of the pathology of atherosclerosis in the UK have died. They include Theo Crawford, Jack Duguid, John French, John Poole and Colin Adams.

Amazingly, in the text of Florey's first edition in 1954, there is no mention of arteriosclerosis as a discrete entity and none of cholesterol. But in the second edition of his textbook in 1958, there is a new chapter by John French entitled 'Atherosclerosis'. In this there is a full account of the infiltration of lipids from the blood. He wrote:

> The lipid composition of the tissue fluid is the factor, which determines the overall severity of tissue changes. The important factor which leads to clinical symptoms in atherosclerosis is thrombosis... The conclusion originally drawn from [animal feeding] experiments was that an

[50] Kohn (1957, 1970). Professor Jim Kohn, Queen Mary's Hospital, Roehampton, produced a number of eletrophoretic techniques, which have been the cornerstone of haemoglobinopathy testing for several decades.

[51] Professor Vincent Marks wrote: 'The drug was candicidin, a polyene macrolide antibiotic that was discovered by Nobel laureate S A Waksman in 1953 at Rutgers University. It reduced the size and cholesterol content of the prostate of elderly dogs used in toxicological studies and led to its hypocholesterolaemic properties being discovered in the late 1960s [Schaffner and Gordon (1968)] and our investigations in the early 1970s.' Note on draft transcript, 16 February 2006.

> abnormally high concentration of cholesterol in the blood was the significant factor in causing the fatty intimal lesions. There is increasing evidence that the severity of the lesions [are] related more closely to the relative proportions of the different plasma lipids.[52]

John French's account was exemplary and ahead of its time. Neville Woolf will now take up the theme.

Professor Neville Woolf: I first became interested in atherosclerosis, probably for the same reason that Barry Lewis and Gerry Shaper did, because I grew up in South Africa where you had to be a really crass observer not to notice that there was as much coronary disease among the white population as anywhere else in the world, but virtually none in the African population. In all the years I spent as a pathologist in Cape Town, I never carried out a post-mortem examination on an African who had CHD and it was only many years later in Britain that I did my first post mortem on an African migrant who had had coronary thrombosis. Round about the same time, Ancel Keys paid a visit to South Africa and he and the late Brian Bronte-Stewart, the first director of the rather short-lived MRC unit in Glasgow [Atheroma Research Unit, 1962–67], did some work together and showed how one could modify plasma cholesterol levels, not only by changing the lipid quantity of the diet, but also the lipid quality, so that if one substituted polyunsaturated fatty acids in the form of sunflower seed oil for animal fats, there was a significant decline in the plasma cholesterol.[53]

When I came to Britain in 1959 there was a comparative lull in the pathological field so far as the atherosclerotic lesion was concerned and I was lucky enough to get a PhD studentship with the late Theo Crawford, who himself had been considerably influenced by John Duguid's descriptive accounts of atherosclerotic plaques and of the contribution that mural thrombi could make to the actual volume of those plaques. The trouble was that it was almost impossible to identify platelets in atherosclerotic lesions reliably, unless they were pretty fresh, and the staining methods that we used for fibrin were somewhat capricious. I was asked by Theo Crawford to try to apply the fairly recently described Coons fluorescent antibody method to the study of atherosclerosis.[54] In that year with my colleague Kelvin Carstairs, we made reasonably pure antibodies

---

[52] French (1958): 376, 369. He remarked that it was impossible to state specifically the cause of atherosclerosis (page 358).

[53] Bronte-Stewart *et al.* (1955); Anderson *et al.* (1956). See also Bronte-Stewart (1965).

[54] See Glossary, page 140.

to fibrin and to platelets.[55] Monoclonal antibodies didn't exist at that time and, of course, it was impossible to buy antibodies commercially; we had to make them ourselves and then conjugate them for ourselves. I have vivid memories of making the organ powders that one needed to get rid of the unconjugated dye. In the laboratory it looked as if there had been an elephant with diarrhoea, with piles of liver puree on the floor. Be that as it may, we did succeed in identifying antigen in these lesions. What was quite interesting, so far as the results using antifibrin antibody were concerned, was that there seemed to be two basic patterns in which these antigens appeared. The first was a more or less diffuse staining of the intima, which at higher resolution could be seen as dot-like areas of fluorescence, whereas in many other areas there were solid bars of fluorescent material that lay roughly parallel to the endothelial surface. When we used an antiplatelet antibody on these same lesions, the platelet antigen co-localized with these bar-like areas within the atherosclerotic plaque. We drew the conclusion, rightly or wrongly, that the bar-like pattern of fibrin deposition represented episodes of mural thrombosis [thrombosis located on the artery wall] and that these thrombi had been covered over by new connective tissue (see Figure 3).

One of the major objections that had always been raised against a contribution of thrombosis to the growth of atherosclerotic plaques was this question: 'How could a thrombus be present within the depths of the plaque cap?' I always used to think of it in terms of burial customs; if somebody is dead, you dig a hole, and then you deposit him at the bottom, and cover it up again. Now I thought that was only one way of burying someone. The other way, which Anglo Saxons used, was to place the deceased person on the ground and cover him. Of course, that's exactly what happens in the artery wall where the presence of thrombus excites the formation of new connective tissue through the medium of proliferating smooth muscle. What was also interesting in a study that we did in 1972, was that we looked at every single, intact plaque in the aortas of patients who had either died from coronary disease or had died from something else. Interestingly enough, those who had had coronary thrombosis showed a much greater number of the aortic plaques with the so-called thrombotic pattern than did the others. It looked as if there were highly significant local factors in coronary thrombosis to which I will allude in a moment, but nevertheless there were some general pro-thrombotic changes in the patients who died of coronary disease.

---

[55] Carstairs *et al.* (1964).

Some of you will remember, of course, that at that time the question of whether thrombosis had anything to do with acute coronary events at all was a highly controversial matter: the British pathologists taking a 'pro' position and the American pathologists taking a distinctly 'anti' position. It was in this particular field that my late colleague Michael Davies,[56] whose early death all of us regret so much, was particularly important, and to which he made particular contributions. Largely as a result of his early studies, there is no doubt now that patients who die with acute coronary disease die with thrombosis, which is related to injury of the plaque cap. In the 1970s Michael Davies described two major forms of plaque cap injury – deep injury or plaque disruption, which counts for about 75 per cent of major coronary thromboses and superficial injury.[57] It's interesting, also perhaps salutary, to think that he obtained his results by the simplest of technical methods, but what he did contribute was a tremendous degree of energy and patience, asking simple questions in a simple way but in very great detail. I think this is a real contribution from pathology to our understanding of what happens in acute coronary events.

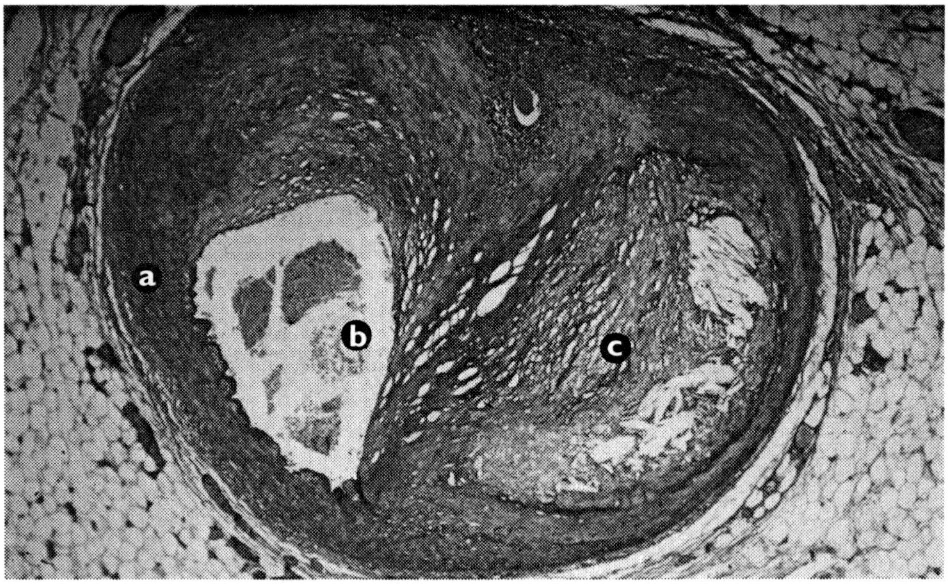

Figure 3: Photomicrograph of a transverse section through a coronary artery [x 35, *c.* 1970]. The photograph shows an eccentric plaque with a lipid-rich pool (c) covered by dark-stained collagen-rich neo-intima.[58] a: intima; b: lumen; c: plaque.

[56] Corbishley and Burke (2003). See also Davies (1992); Lendon *et al.* (1992).

[57] Davies *et al.* (1976, 1994).

[58] Lendrum (1949).

Lastly, there was the question that if acute coronary events are preceded by a plaque injury, what are the circumstances that underlie that injury? Here, again, I would like to pay tribute to Mike Davies for his work in this area, where he measured the volume of plaques and in particular of the atheromatous pool in those plaques and found that there was a critical volume of pool which if exceeded meant that the patient was very likely to have splitting of the cap and consequent thrombosis.[59] This was about 40 per cent of the plaque volume. This was accompanied by a comparative paucity of smooth muscles and a marked increase – which wasn't relative but an absolute increase – in lipid-laden macrophages [Figure 4]. Mike brought us to the threshold of the current era, where he was interested in the role of inflammatory mediators in bringing about pool formation and cap necrosis.

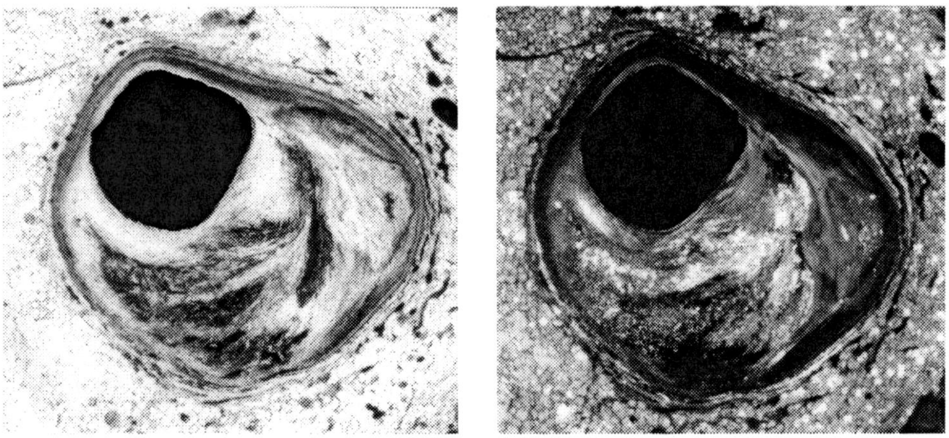

4a. Unstained section photographed by normal transmitted light.

4b. The same section in polarized light revealing the distribution of cholesterol crystals, which shine like stars.

Figure 4: Frozen section of an atherosclerotic coronary artery. The lumen is occupied by opaque injection medium [x 15, 1953].[60] From Fulton (1965): 237.

[59] Davies and Thomas (1985); Davies (1996).

[60] Dr Bill Fulton wrote: 'In contrast to paraffin sections, in which cholesterol and neutral fat are totally removed in the processing, they are preserved in the frozen section. Cholesterol tends to be deposited mainly in the amorphous material in the plaque. The distribution of cholesterol is positively demonstrated in scintillating fashion by polarized light (4b). This is an example of a complex atherosclerotic plaque with layered crescentric structure.' Letter to Professor Michael Oliver, 17 January 2006.

Oliver: Now I am sure Elspeth Smith will have a view about the infiltration of the arterial wall.

Dr Elspeth Smith: First of all I would like to remind people that the earliest study of atherosclerosis was by Anitschkov in 1913, who fed cholesterol to rabbits.[61] But more recently, we became interested in lipoprotein studies in the 1950s when Gofman had already produced some of his results.[62] There were Oliver and Boyd, there was Fredrickson's group, and Dangerfield and I, and all developed the electrophoresis of lipoproteins by paper and staining with Sudan Black.[63] During the 1950s, there were sporadic studies on the lipids in the artery wall, but in the 1960s we began to study them in detail. In my case this was partly brought about by the fact that the pre-β lipoprotein seemed to be particularly associated with coronary disease and we were wondering what differences there were in the lipid content of the different lipoprotein bands in the artery wall. In the 1960s we started a fairly detailed and systematic study of the artery wall, and the main groups involved were Böttcher in Leiden, and my own group working on humans, and Adams, Gresham, Howard, and Bowyer, working on animals in this country.[64] We found – in fact we disagreed strongly with Böttcher on this – that it was necessary to isolate intima and media, normal intima from lesions, and different sorts of plaques, because they all were analysed and produced quite different results. Meanwhile, gas chromatography was developed and this enabled us to study the different cholesterol ester fatty acids. It became clear that the extracellular perifibrous lipids in normal intima and in fibrous-type plaques was closely related to LDL or β-lipoprotein, whereas in the fatty streaks it was completely different and the fatty acid was almost entirely oleic acid; the fatty acid in the extracellular lipid was mainly linoleic acid, which agreed with the LDL.[65] By the mid-1960s, I think Woolf and Pilkington did some immunological studies on lipoproteins, and Haust, and also Walton, certainly showed that they could demonstrate immunofluorescence of LDL in intimas.[66] That led us to try to measure the amount of lipoprotein in intima. Actually we

---

[61] Anitschkov and Chalatow (1913).

[62] For example, Gofman *et al.* (1952).

[63] Oliver and Boyd (1955); Dangerfield and Smith (1955); Fredrickson *et al.* (1967).

[64] See, for example, Adams *et al.* (1963); Smith (1965); Böttcher (1967); Howard *et al.* (1972).

[65] Smith *et al.* (1967).

[66] See, for example, Walton and Scott (1964); Woolf and Pilkington (1965); Haust *et al.* (1967).

developed a very satisfactory method of analysing little bits of tissue put into an electrophoresis gel and then run directly into antibodies. In that way we got lipoproteins without the possible damage that occurred in trying to extract them. That showed us in about 1970 that there was a direct correlation between serum and intimal LDL in normal intima.

In the 1970s Goldstein and Brown's description of a receptor for LDL was published and many people jumped on to the bandwagon on receptors of one sort or another.[67] One of the questions that arose was the question of permeability of endothelium, and it was held very firmly that the endothelium would not allow large particles such as LDL to enter the intima, and yet we found that the amount of lipoprotein was actually greater than the amount of plasma; the concentration was actually greater than in plasma.[68] This was also corroborated by Hoff and co-workers in the US.[69] There was considerable argument as to how it went in.

About 1976 Werthessen and co-workers showed that the usual sort of standard cholesterol that was used for feeding to rabbits was actually highly oxidized and that if you fed them absolutely pure cholesterol it had a very much less atherogenic effect.[70] That was another thing that was to run and run, particularly with the demonstration of scavenger receptors in macrophages.[71] One of the most fascinating things that we found was that in areas containing fat-filled cells, although there was an enormously high cholesterol-only content, the amount of lipoproteins there was extremely low, and this led to a question of receptors, the macrophage receptors and what happened.[72] I still firmly believe that macrophages are oxidizing their own lipoprotein, taking it up in the oxidized lipoprotein (LP) receptors, rather than a general oxidation. Well, the system of the permeability of the endothelium was finally solved by Simionescu, who showed that there was a vesicular transport and that all the large particles went into the intima through vesicular transport and accumulated there.[73] We started

---

[67] Goldstein and Brown (1977).

[68] Smith and Slater (1972); Smith and Staples (1980, 1982).

[69] Hoff *et al.* (1977).

[70] Imai *et al.* (1976).

[71] Henriksen *et al.* (1981).

[72] Smith and Ashall (1983).

[73] Simionescu (1980).

using the interstitial fluid rather than the whole intima and we found that the concentrations of LDL in interstitial fluid were consistently about twice the plasma concentration. This could really only be explained by the idea of being carried in by vesicular transport. It was then blocked by the internal elastic lamina and it was only when it had built up to a really high concentration that it went out again through the endothelium. Since then I don't think there has been so much work on endothelial lipids themselves.

Professor Gustav Born: Thank you very much, Michael, for letting me make a short contribution that follows on well from Elspeth's. Having done what we could to help to elucidate the platelet contribution to arterial obstruction, notably coronary thrombosis and stroke, it was natural to turn to the atherosclerosis contribution, the subject of this Witness Seminar.[74] As well as working on plaque fissure in the late 1980s and early 1990s,[75] we turned to what Elspeth has been talking about, namely the transfer of LDL from the blood into the artery walls. The Steins in Jerusalem had followed the transport of radio-labelled plasma protein into rat aortic walls by autoradiography; and the Simionescus had demonstrated binding, endocytosis and trancytosis of LDL in arterial endothelium using electron microscopy.[76] Goldstein and Brown established the LDL concentration in the plasma as presumptively the most important determinant of the rate of atherogenesis: the more you have the sooner and the worse is the disease.[77]

We asked the question, whether there are any other determinants of LDL flux into artery walls? In the course of about ten years' work we produced convincing experimental evidence that the arterial accumulations of LDL and of fibrinogen – another atherogenic plasma protein very different in size and properties from LDL – are very similarly influenced by structural and hormonal factors.[78] A most important structural determinant turned out to be the density of free negative

---

[74] Born (2002, 2003); Reynolds and Tansey (eds) (2005).

[75] Richardson *et al.* (1989).

[76] Stein *et al.* (1973); Vasile *et al.* (1983).

[77] Goldstein and Brown (1977). They received the Nobel Prize in Physiology or Medicine in 1985 for their work in identifying the low-density lipoprotein receptor pathway, the mechanism controlling how the body's cells obtain cholesterol. They also determined how an inherited defect in this pathway, occurring in the disease familial hypercholesterolaemia, can lead to atherosclerosis, a disease resulting in cholesterol-clogged arteries. See http://nobelprize.org/medicine/laureates/1985/index.html (visited 2 November 2005).

[78] For a review, see Born *et al.* (2003).

charges on arterial endothelium. The lumenal surface is covered by a layer rich in glycoproteins which extend acidic sialate groups into the flowing blood plasma. When intact, anaesthetized rabbits' and rats' large arteries were briefly perfused with the enzyme neuraminidase to remove these sialic acids selectively, the subsequent flux of LDL from plasma into arterial walls was accelerated. This effect being demonstrable in two mammalian species, one imagines that something similar also happens in humans. I am now working with Michael Frenneaux, Professor of Cardiology in Birmingham, to see if we can obtain such evidence with material ethically obtained from patients undergoing bypass surgery. As vascular endothelia have extraordinarily high negative charge densities, and as circulating LDL is also negatively charged, the most likely explanation is simply electrostatic repulsion.[79] Although endothelia do have some high affinity LDL receptors, all the evidence so far is that the entry of LDL into endothelial caveoli and from there into arterial intima is by diffusion. The exact mechanism(s) of these processes have still to be worked out.

Another most interesting finding had to do with endogenous pressor agents, very relevant, of course, because hypertension is a major risk factor for the clinical manifestations of atherosclerotic diseases such as MI and stroke. In a series of papers we reported evidence on the acceleration of the flux of LDL and of fibrinogen into arterial walls induced by endogenous mediators. Infused adrenaline and noradrenaline accelerate the uptake of LDL in rabbit carotids and rat aortae *in vivo*.[80] The experimental procedures were entirely different in the two species, so that the results corroborated each other. Striking confirmatory evidence was the opposite effect in animals treated with reserpine, which removes endogenous catecholamines and which reduced the uptake of LDL by arterial walls. Other means of raising blood pressure had similar effects, viz. cortisol plus sodium chloride and, most interestingly, so did the *in vivo* inhibition by L-NAME [N(G)-nitro-L-arginine methylester] of nitric oxide production. Conversely, when nitric oxide production by cultured endothelial cells (HUVEC, human umbilical vein endothelial cells) was increased LDL uptake was diminished – more evidence that nitric oxide is antiatherogenic; an important effect demonstrated also by others using different techniques. Together, the experiments strongly suggest a relationship between blood pressure and atherogenesis. These experimental observations are now also being followed up clinically in Birmingham.

---

[79] Born and Palinski (1985).

[80] For review, see Born *et al.* (2003).

Oliver: One of the major contributors is Gordon Lowe. He took on the thrombosis theme from Jack Duguid, pathologist in Newcastle in 1953–4, who identified the importance of thrombus. Can you take us a little bit further forward?

Professor Gordon Lowe: Moving from the solid phase of thrombus to the fluid phase: haemostasis laboratories, such as our own in Glasgow – which was set up in the 1950s by Stuart Douglas and George McNicol – were looking at the degree to which lipids might provoke thrombosis in circulating blood, looking at platelets, coagulation and fibrinolysis.[81] I will just give you a minute on each of these three.

In the 1970s platelets were championed as Gus Born and John O'Brien invented platelet aggregation techniques.[82] Aspirin was shown to be an antiplatelet drug, and we all know from trials done over the past 30 years that aspirin and other antiplatelet agents are effective treatment for the acute coronary syndromes and also in prevention. Platelets are quite difficult to study, but in the 1970s a variety of techniques became available so that we could look at platelet function *in vivo*. That was by looking at circulating platelet aggregates, plasma levels of platelet release products such as β-thromboglobulin, and urinary measurement of thromboxane metabolites. Studies by several groups, including our own, showed that patients with congenital hypercholesterolaemia, but also people with acquired hyperlipidaemia, have activated platelets.[83] Subsequent experimental work in the 1980s and 1990s shows that this was because oxidized LDL, which Elspeth mentioned, but also VLDL in particular, altered membranes in the platelets of such patients, and indeed, incubation of normal platelets with these lipid fractions could result in platelet activation.

Moving from platelets to coagulation, it's important to recognize that coagulation takes place on the surface of activated cells, not only platelets but also endothelial cells and monocytes, and with the development of vascular biology over the past 30 years, studies of isolated cells have shown that lipids and lipoproteins – again especially oxidized LDL – activated not only platelets but also endothelial cells and monocytes, changing them from a resting state into a procoagulant phase. In particular activated endothelial cells and monocytes produce tissue

[81] See, for example, McNicol and Douglas (1964).

[82] There is some dispute over the invention and development of these techniques, see Reynolds and Tansey (eds) (2005): 6–10, 23.

[83] Lowe *et al.* (1980).

factor, which interacts with coagulation factor VII to initiate blood coagulation through the tissue factor pathway. The observation that increased blood lipids activate clotting is, in fact, rather old, it goes back to the early 1950s when H W Fullerton and colleagues studied the effects of postprandial lipidaemia on clotting times.[84] And in particular, when the Russell viper venom that came from that common reptile was added to plasma it was particularly sensitive in showing that there was an effect. My old boss Colin Prentice told me it was suggested that this observation was only relevant to people who ate a fatty meal before walking into the jungle and being bitten by a snake. [Laughter.] But little did the critics know that the Russell viper venom is a specific activator of the tissue factor pathway and this early observation highlighted the potential role of this pathway in thrombosis, which is now accepted as the main way in which blood coagulation is activated. Over the last 25 years the work of Professors Tom Meade and George Miller here in London has established that factor VII is associated with coronary risk, and again is associated with both congenital and acquired hyperlipidaemias.[85] Furthermore, they showed that one of the fibrates, gemfibrozil, reduced not only triglyceride but also reduced factor VII as well as levels of prothrombin activation peptide, which indicates a reduction of thrombin generation *in vivo*.[86] And then finally, in the Thrombosis Prevention Trial of warfarin and aspirin organized by Tom Meade that reported a few years ago, warfarin, which effectively lowers factor VII levels, was shown to be an effective component in primary prevention of CHD, especially in fatal events, in this factorial trial.[87] In a recent collaborative substudy in this trial between London and Glasgow, we showed that such efficacy in preventing fatal MI was critically dependent on achieving a reduction in thrombin generation as shown by activation markers. And also thereby achieving a reduction in turnover of fibrin as shown by a reduction in plasma levels of fibrin D-dimer, which in studies from our laboratory over the past 15 years has been established as a significant predictor of coronary risk.[88]

What about the role of lipids in fibrinolysis? Again it was Tom Meade who published a study showing that a prolonged blood clot lysis time, which

---

[84] Fullerton *et al.* (1953).

[85] Miller *et al.* (1985); Miller (1999).

[86] Wilkes *et al.* (1992).

[87] Medical Research Council's General Practice Research Framework (1998).

[88] MacCallum *et al.* (2004).

indicates reduced fibrinolytic potential, was associated with coronary risk in a prospective study.[89] Previous work in the 1960s by Fearnley and Chakrabarti in Gloucester had established that hyperlipidaemia was also associated with prolonged blood clot lysis time.[90] And then in the 1980s the molecular basis of this connection was established by identification of antiplasmin; tissue plasminogen activator as the main enzyme in endogenous fibrinolysis and then by characterization of plasminogen activator inhibitor as the major fibrinolytic inhibitor.[91] Subsequently, very active epidemiological studies, particularly from Irène Juhan-Vague in France, have established that it is increased levels of these fibrinolytic inhibitors that are associated with hyperlipidaemia, particularly triglyceride in the Metabolic Syndrome as well as coronary risk.[92]

Back in the 1950s, Tage Astrup in Denmark hypothesized that there was a physiological balance between coagulation and fibrinolysis, and that hyperlipidaemia and other risk factors alter the balance in favour of increased coagulation and decreased fibrinolysis and that would favour thrombosis.[93] In the 1980s, Hymie Nossel in New York produced radioimmunoassays of fibrinopeptide A as a marker of thrombin activity *in vivo*, and a fragment of fibrin that was a measure of plasmin lysis. He hypothesized that if you measured blood levels of these two activation products to obtain a ratio, this would be a balance between coagulation and fibrinolysis. David Wood and I performed a study in the late 1980s in which we studied people from Edinburgh, shipped the samples to Glasgow and measured them. We showed two basic things, that hyperlipidaemia would unbalance coagulation and fibrinolysis; and also that collaboration between Glasgow and Edinburgh was occasionally possible.[94]

Oliver: To end this session on pathology, it should be recorded that there were three atheroma regression studies conducted in the UK in the 1980s and 1990s. These demonstrated that some degree of regression is possible with sustained reduction of raised plasma cholesterol concentrations.

---

[89] Meade *et al.* (1993).

[90] Chakrabarti *et al.* (1968).

[91] Lowe *et al.* (1982).

[92] Juhan-Vague *et al.* (2003).

[93] Astrup (1956); Gaffney *et al.* (1999).

[94] Lowe *et al.* (1991).

In 1983, a group from St Thomas' reported the effect of plasma lipid reduction on the progression of femoral atherosclerosis in 24 hyperlipidaemic patients with stable intermittent claudication.[95] The patients were randomly assigned to treatment and usual-care groups, the former receiving dietary advice and cholestyramine, nicotinic acid, or clofibrate depending on their lipoprotein phenotype. Biplanar arteriography was performed when the study began and after a mean period of 19 months. Angiograms were assessed visually, with observer blinding, and by computerized image analysis. Therapy reduced mean plasma total cholesterol by 25 per cent, mean low density lipoprotein (LDL) cholesterol by 28 per cent, and mean plasma triglycerides by 45 per cent. Significantly fewer arterial segments showed detectable progression of atherosclerosis in the treatment group. In both groups, changes in edge irregularity index were directly related to plasma LDL cholesterol concentration.[96] This study was the first randomized controlled trial of its type and provided evidence that effective treatment of hyperlipidaemia favourably influences the natural history of symptomatic peripheral atherosclerosis.

In 1992, using quantitative coronary angiography, the St Thomas' Hospital trial (STARS) reported the effects over 39 months of dietary intervention in 90 hypercholesterolaemic men with CHD.[97] Dietary change alone retarded overall progression and increased overall regression of coronary artery disease. Diet plus cholestyramine was additionally associated with a net increase in coronary lumen diameter.

In 1994, a multicentre antiatheroma trial (MAAS), in which Gilbert Thompson and I took part, showed that simvastatin had a similar effect on lesions in the coronary arteries: 381 men with CHD were randomized to simvastatin and placebo pills.[98] Using three serial coronary angiograms over four years, measured by quantitative techniques, the effect of sustained lowering of LDL by 31 per cent reduced progression of lesions. Actual regression of coronary lesions was slow but became evident after four years of simvastatin treatment.

Dr Arthur Hollman: Just a very brief comment about thrombosis and the coronary arteries. I don't think we should pass on without referring to Bill

---

[95] Duffield *et al.* (1983).

[96] See Glossary, page 141, for the edge-irregularity index used in the St Thomas' Atherosclerosis Regression Study (STARS).

[97] Watts *et al.* (1992).

[98] Multicentre Anti-Atheroma Study (MAAS) (1994).

Fulton in Glasgow.[99] I will be very brief. Patients admitted with an MI were injected with a radioactive substance. Those that died had their coronary thrombosis examined and he showed that the radioactivity had accumulated in the thrombosis that killed them. There was no doubt that the thrombus preceded the MI. A fine bit of tuned experimentation, but I doubt whether it would get through a clinical trial today.

Oliver: I had asked Joan Slack to come in here, but unfortunately her husband is sufficiently ill for her to telephone two days ago to say that she would not be able to come, but Joan's paper in the *Journal of Medical Genetics* in 1968, on the mode of inheritance of xanthomata in 55 families, was probably the first publication on genetic inheritance in the UK.[100] Joan then produced a paper in the *Lancet* on ischaemic heart disease in familial hyperlipoproteinaemia, based on the same 55 families.[101] Possibly the first observation about the genetic susceptibility to ischaemic heart disease was by Gertler and White in the US. In 1954 they published a monograph entitled 'Coronary heart disease in young adults'.[102] In this they described 100 cases under the age of 40, of which 97 were males. They did not produce information about lipoproteins. Geoffrey Rose also recorded the importance of familial clustering, although not specifically related to hypercholesterolaemia.[103]

Professor Steve Humphries: I personally am sad that Joan Slack isn't here, because I have been looking forward to seeing her again. I met her 20-odd years ago when I first started in this field. We talked quite a lot about her papers. She started publishing in the 1960s, on various inborn errors of metabolism. Between 1970 and 1980 she published 14 papers in collaboration with people like Nick Myant whom we have heard about; June Lloyd, Institute of Child Health, who sadly had a stroke about ten years ago; and Arvin Heiberg in Norway, who showed the links with Käre Berg and some of their Scandinavian colleagues,[104] all of whom were interested in this issue: what is the relative contribution of

---

[99] Fulton (1993). See also discussion on pages 18–19, and Figure 3.

[100] Slack and Evans (1966); Slack and Nevin (1968); Nevin and Slack (1968). See page 14 for a discussion of Müller's study of 17 Oslo families [Müller (1939)].

[101] Slack (1969).

[102] Gertler and White (1954).

[103] Rose (1964).

[104] See, for example, Heiberg and Berg (1976).

family history to heart disease, particularly with a focus on lipids?[105] The paper that Michael mentioned was published by David Patterson at UCL, who is still working at the Whittington Hospital, in the *Lancet* in 1972.[106] They came up with the estimate that roughly 5 per cent of men who had a heart attack under the age of 55 had this pattern of type IIa hypercholesterolaemia [elevated LDL cholesterol] when you looked at their relatives, and this estimate of about 5 per cent was confirmed in the series of three papers that came out in the US in 1973, published in the *Journal of Clinical Investigation* from Arno Motulsky, Joe Goldstein and others.[107] I am quite interested to know whether it is still the case that 5 per cent of young MI cases have this IIa pattern or whether that has changed. I am not aware of any data about that.

I am going to say a couple more things about hypercholesterolaemia, but one of the genetic determinants of plasma lipids which I would like to mention is the gene coding for the apolipoprotein, apoE. Looking round the room, I think that about half of us have published a paper with apoE in it, so it is a popular gene to work on. From my understanding, it was possible, probably in the late 1960s or early 1970s, to use isoelectric focusing gels to determine that there were three common isoforms known as E3, E2 and E4. There is a very strong and consistent association between the apoE phenotype (and genotype) and plasma lipids and risk of heart disease. It has quite a small effect on lipids, but because it's rather a common variant, it actually has a modest but quite consistent effect on CHD

---

[105] Dr Nick Myant wrote: 'Joan Slack routinely saw patients at the weekly morning sessions of the Hammersmith Lipid Clinic. At the end of the Clinic she always came up to my office, where we ate a sandwich lunch and discussed such topics as population genetics (Slack was one of my genetics mentors). We were both interested in the contribution of genetic factors to hypercholesterolaemia in the general UK population – in particular the possible contribution from heterozygous FH. The difficulty was that we had no idea of the frequency of FH heterozygotes in the UK. One day early in 1971 it occurred to me that if one made an uneducated guess as to the maximum probable number of FH homozygotes in the UK (I think I suggested 40), one could estimate an upper limit for the frequency of FH heterozygotes using the Hardy–Weinberg equation for the frequencies of the three genotypes at a diallelic locus. I put this to Joan Slack at our next lunch meeting and she said she would discuss it with Cedric Carter, her boss in the MRC Clinical Genetics Unit. The upshot was that a day or two later, Carter wrote a joint letter to the *Lancet* (on his way home by train, so he claimed) in which we said that the incidence of heterozygous FH in the UK was unlikely to be more than 0.5 per cent [Carter *et al.* (1971)]. As the years went by it became obvious that we had overestimated the number of homozygotes in the UK. In 1976 [Myant (1990a): 405] we made another estimate based on a lower number of homozygotes, suggesting that the frequency of heterozygotes in the UK was about 1:500. Crude though these estimates were, they allowed us to conclude that only a very small fraction of people with hypercholesterolaemia in the general population are carriers of the FH mutation.' Letter to Mrs Lois Reynolds, 16 February 2006.

[106] Patterson and Slack (1972).

[107] Goldstein *et al.* (1973a and b); Hazzard *et al.* (1973).

risk as described by Bob Mahley in the US; Gerd Utermann in Germany; Forbes Robertson in Aberdeen; Jean Davignon in Canada; and Charlie Sing in the US.[108] I think it is an important gene, and definitely one that shouldn't be overlooked.

There are two things I want to say about the LDL receptor: the first is the issue of the frequency of heterozygous familial hypercholesterolaemia (FH) in the UK, and I was hoping that Nick Myant and Joan Slack would be here to confirm this story. I imagine that there was a conversation where it was realized that you could estimate the frequency of heterozygous FH if you knew how many homozygotes there were. And, of course, homozygous FH presents in childhood with very early demonstration of coronary artery disease and clear signs of cholesterol deposits in the skin and tendons, so essentially all paediatric cases would be identified. It was realized that deconvoluting the Hardy–Weinberg equation where q is the frequency of the mutation carrier and p is the frequency of the noncarrier, $p^2 + 2pq + q^2 = 1$, and so if you know q^2 you can actually work out 2pq. My imagination is that Joan and Nick and June Lloyd and others were sitting around the table having a cup of tea and someone suddenly realized that you could do this if you knew how many homozygotes there were. June was looking after some cases and Gil Thompson was looking after others and suddenly they came up with a figure, added a 'fudge factor' for the ones that had died, divided by the population of Britain and came up with the estimate that the frequency of homozygous FH is 1 in one million, from which you could work out that the carrier is 1 in 500. Now maybe that is completely wrong, I don't know if there's anyone around the table here who can comment.[109]

---

[108] See, for example, Utermann *et al.* (1975); Pitas *et al.* (1979); Robertson and Cumming (1985); Sing and Davignon (1985).

[109] Professor Steve Humphries wrote: 'My second comment about the LDL receptor was about an incident that occurred in 1985 when we first started working on the LDL receptor gene in FH patients in the UK. Dave Russell, working with Brown and Goldstein, had very kindly sent us his human LDLR probe and, using Southern blotting methods, we had identified the first common polymorphism of the gene. This enabled us to track the defective LDLR gene through families, which, of course, meant that it would be possible to use this as a DNA diagnostic tool in children. I was working with Professor Bob Williamson at St Mary's Hospital, London, at the time, and we collaborated with David Galton, Mary Seed, Victor Wynn and others, showed that diagnosis was possible in two families, and prepared a manuscript which we hoped to submit to the *Lancet* [Humphries *et al.* (1985)]. I asked Gil Thompson to have a look at it for an expert opinion before I sent it in. He replied saying this was very interesting and hoped that the *Lancet* would like it, but he very much doubted it would ever become of widespread use in clinical practice. Here we are almost 20 years on and I am afraid Gil is still right about it not being in widespread use, although several of us around the table would hope that, if we can make the DNA methodology much cheaper, it might still have a place in helping give an unambiguous diagnosis of FH in families where lipid levels do not give a clear answer.' Note on draft transcript, 7 September 2005.

Professor Hugh Tunstall-Pedoe: I can answer that because I attended a meeting at the Hammersmith Hospital, London, in the 1970s which was convened to discuss exactly that question. British lipidologists had got together to discuss the number of cases of homozygous familial hypercholesterolaemia that they knew about in the UK. There was an impression that it was more common than it actually was. Each of them was aware of a handful of cases and they thought they would multiply them *pro rata*, but it turned out that they had a lot of cases in common, so many of the cases they were talking about were the same and far fewer than they had imagined.[110]

Oliver: James Scott, would you like to take up the theme of genetics?

Professor James Scott: We did molecular genetics rather than genetics. In 1970 when introns were discovered in globin genes, I went to see Chris Booth, and my mentor Tim Peters, and said, 'I want to do this molecular biology.' They sent me to see Sydney Brenner, who, among others, suggested that I might join Bill Rutter in Biochemistry at the University of California in San Francisco. It was at this time quite difficult for a jobbing, trainee physician to get money to train in molecular genetics. In the end, I managed to get a fellowship from the European Molecular Biology Organization (EMBO). After two-and-a-half years with Bill Rutter working on growth factors, I came to the conclusion that I wanted to work on something other than growth control and cancer, and to do something that was highly clinically relevant. Just after this time, and after writing the Fellowship to come back to London, Steve Humphries came to see me in California and we chatted about what we both might do in London. Initially we pursued the smaller apolipoprotein genes and had a number of publications. However, at the Gordon Conference in 1984 I formed the view that we should have a crack at apolipoprotein B (apoB).[111]

At this stage nobody even had a clue how large the protein was. It was variously estimated as being between 20 kDa [thousand Daltons] and 3 million kDa in size. The problem with apoB is that once it is delipidated it behaves like chewing gum on a hot summer's day – it is virtually impossible to get a good protein sequence. I then came across Howard Morris and Ann Dell working at

---

[110] Professor Hugh Tunstall-Pedoe wrote: 'Using the Hardy–Weinberg equation, the projected prevalence of heterozygous familial hypercholesterolaemia was correspondingly lower and their projection at that time of 1 in 500 of the population is an estimate that I do not think has ever subsequently been revised.' Note on draft transcript, 8 January 2006. See note 105. See also Glossary, page 142.

[111] The Gordon Conference on Lipid Metabolism, Meriden, NH, July 1984.

Imperial College. They had made a series of developments in mass spectroscopy, which could be used for protein sequencing, including, unusually, the carboxyl terminal of proteins, providing the protein could be solubilized in high concentrations of SDS (sodium dodecyl sulphate). I therefore went to see Chris Booth, then head of the MRC Clinical Research Centre at Northwick Park Hospital, London, and said: 'Look, we haven't got the technology that we need for this, but will you give us £10 000 so that Howard Morris can do this in his company, called M-SCAN?'[112] After some thought, Chris agreed. We went off to get bits of apoB protein sequence and this facilitated the cloning of the extremely large apoB cDNA. To get more of this we contacted Bob Mahley, head of Gladstone Laboratories at the University of California, San Francisco.[113] Somewhat to Bob's angst, we also teamed up with Jake Lusis at the University of California, Los Angeles. Together the three groups stitched the carboxyl terminal sequence of apoB and published this in *Science*, and then pulled the whole sequence together and published this in *Nature*.[114] At the time apoB was the largest protein to have been sequenced with a molecular weight of over one half million. It had 4536 amino acids.

At the same time, we were very serious about the origins of apolipoprotein B48 and thought that this had to be something peculiar. While we were dealing with cDNA, Bob Mahley and his colleagues had been dealing with the gene in parallel. The gene structure was published in the *Journal of Biological Chemistry*.[115] We found that the gene was grossly asymmetrical, and that there was one huge 3' exon encoding half the protein. We pinpointed the origins of the carboxyl terminal of apoB48, using expressed clones and monoclonal antibodies, and then pulled out all the cDNA clones from this region in several human cDNA libraries. A couple of months later I was talking with Joe Goldstein who said: 'I bet there's something odd going on to generate apoB48.' I agreed: 'There are a series of stop codons at that site where the protein ends,' and he laughed. But about two months later we were able to submit to *Nature* that in humans and rabbits there was indeed a stop codon that coincided with the end of apoB48, but that this was not encoded in the genome. A genomically encoded C was transposed to U in the RNA, converting a glutamine to a stop translation codon.

---

[112] Operating in 2006 as M-SCAN Mass Spectrometry Research and Training Centre, Silwood Park, Ascot SL5 7PZ.

[113] Mahley and Innerarity (1978); Innerarity and Mahley (1978).

[114] Knott *et al.* (1985, 1986).

[115] Blackhart *et al.* (1986).

We postulated that there was a site-specific cytidine deamination of the RNA, and that it was due to editing of the mRNA. Unfortunately, *Nature* turned down the manuscript. Thanks to Peter Rigby we were able to publish this in *Cell*.[116] We found a number of other editing genes in 2002. These turned out to be very interesting, because they edit DNA and are involved in the creation of the antibody diversity, and appear to form an innate mechanism that destroys retroviral genomes.

Oliver: We aren't intending to go beyond 2000.

Booth: May I make a comment about James Scott's work when he was at Northwick Park. I think that directors of institutes don't normally get mixed up in the actual science that many of their science staff do. On this occasion I did. In James' case when he produced this extraordinary story, I went up to Cambridge to see Max Perutz and I showed him James' experiments and asked, 'Is there anything in your molecular model, some little change, that could make this happen?' And he said, 'No.' And in fact I don't think he believed it.

Galton: Most of British lipidology, I think, has lagged way behind the American effort. But there's another first which I think we can put up and that is the first isolation of an apolipoprotein gene by Tito Baralle in Oxford, published I think in 1981.[117] I think it was three weeks before Jan Breslow's publication identifying the same gene and he had found a second one, the apolipoprotein CIII gene at the same locus.[118] I think it was significant that Tito Baralle got there first. Jan Breslow is still a staff member working at the Rockefeller Institute. Tito Baralle left Oxford and is now working in Trieste in northern Italy. [119]

Oliver: Why do we lose our really talented people?

Humphries: I would like to take up the apoAI story for a few minutes. In molecular biology there have been three key developments that have enabled us to study human disease at the DNA level: first there was 'Southern blotting', which was invented in 1975 by Dr Ed Southern, and then, of course, we were able

---

[116] Powell *et al.* (1987).

[117] Shoulders and Baralle (1982).

[118] Zannis *et al.* (1981).

[119] In 2005 Breslow was at the Laboratory of Biochemical Genetics and Metabolism, The Rockefeller University, New York; and Baralle at the International Centre for Genetic Engineering and Biotechnology, Trieste, Italy.

to start looking at human genetic variation, although very slowly.[120] Then came the polymerase chain reaction (PCR), which was invented in 1985 and enabled us to work at least 100 times faster in identifying mutations and screening DNA samples.[121] Then we sprang into this century with the completion of the human genome sequence, which is all the science data that we need to keep us going for the next 20 years.

But the paper that David [Galton] has just mentioned, the cloning of the apoAI gene, enabled David and his colleagues to publish in the *Lancet* in 1983, a milestone paper in my view, looking at the first polymorphism in an apolipoprotein gene.[122] He used the apoAI gene as a probe and found a polymorphic (restriction enzyme cutting) site with the enzyme SstI. The base change creating the polymorphism is not itself functional, but it was associated with hypertriglyceridaemia. They found that the SstI site was more common in a sample of 35 patients than it was in 75 controls. This was all done using Southern blotting and took weeks to produce the data. These days you wouldn't be able to publish such data in a journal of any repute, unless you had ten times, or maybe 100 times those numbers of people. But that was a big experiment in those days. David and his colleagues, Carol Shoulders, Alan Rees and others, speculated that somehow this must mean that apoAI has something to do with triglyceride metabolism. Well, we know now, of course, that they were not correct and that the Sst site was in the end of the apoCIII gene, which is next to the apoAI gene, and that apoCIII has a lot to do with triglyceride metabolism.[123] It is a milestone paper. The interesting thing is that we still don't know, 20 years later, what the molecular mechanism of this effect is, but it is just like apoE, in being a common variant of modest effect on lipid levels and risk. It is also one of the more consistent associations. There are 50–100 papers that have been published where this same observation has been confirmed. In my opinion, it is one of the main pieces of work that came out of the UK in the 1980s.

Oliver: We have to round the session off with a comment from Gilbert Thompson on apheresis.

Thompson: Apheresis, as you all know, means to take away, and it was first done in 1967 by de Gennes and colleagues when they treated a patient with

---

[120] Southern (1975).

[121] Mullis *et al.* (1986); Mullis (1990).

[122] Rees *et al.* (1983).

[123] Rees *et al.* (1985).

homozygous familial hypercholesterolaemia (FH) over a period of three months.[124] They literally took off a bottle of blood, spun it down, removed the plasma and put the cells back; they did this repetitively and called it *traitment heroique*. After three months they gave up and I am afraid the patient soon died, like so many homozygotes used to in those days. Subsequently, the continuous flow blood cell separator was invented at the National Cancer Institute.[125] There was one at the Hammersmith, and I realized the potential of this for undertaking continuous flow plasma exchange. With a blood flow rate of 40ml a minute, over the course of three hours you can exchange 4l or so of a patient's plasma for albumin, which preserves the osmotic pressure and has the advantage that albumin solutions have no cholesterol in them whatsoever. We were able to reduce cholesterol levels by more than 50 per cent in these homozygotes.[126] And in conjunction with Nick Myant and Paul Miller we were able to demonstrate regression of xanthomata in the homozygotes and even obtained some uncontrolled data suggesting that we were getting regression of their atheroma.[127] We were also able to show that the life expectancy of the treated homozygotes was significantly longer than that of their untreated siblings, who obviously had exactly the same defect.[128] So this was a useful addition to the therapeutic armoury which basically had been pretty bare up until plasma exchange came in.

Perhaps I could mention one other aspect of plasma exchange, and that was that, although we usually used it to treat familial hypercholesterolaemia, there was one exception in 1981, a patient with primary biliary cirrhosis and xanthomatous neuropathy.[129] This is an extremely painful condition and you get so much hyperaesthesia that you can't actually turn the key in your own front door lock. She was a patient of Neil McIntyre and Sheila Sherlock. They referred her for plasma exchange, to see if this could alleviate her condition, because it had already been shown by Les Turnberg to be successful in that condition.[130] Anyway we had her over at the Hammersmith, and a friend of

---

[124] de Gennes *et al.* (1967).

[125] See Glossary, page 140.

[126] Thompson *et al.* (1975).

[127] Thompson *et al.* (1980).

[128] Thompson *et al.* (1985).

[129] Thompson (1983).

[130] Turnberg *et al.* (1972).

Neil's who was a pharmacologist, Jonathan Tobert, happened to be over from the US and we got talking.[131] This was about six months after his colleague Alberts had described the cholesterol-lowering potential of lovastatin (originally called mevinolin).[132] Tobert gave me a small supply of lovastatin which we used in conjunction with plasma exchange in this lady and demonstrated that the problem we had previously of a very rapid rebound in cholesterol after plasma exchange could be markedly slowed by inhibiting HMG-CoA reductase at the same time. I think this was probably the first time that a statin had ever been used in Britain. Subsequently I managed to continue to get supplies of lovastatin on a named-patient basis from Merck and we used this on our patients with familial hypercholesterolaemia at the Hammersmith, with considerable benefit to the patients.[133] We continued having this facility from Merck until 1989 when simvastatin became licensed in the UK.[134]

Oliver: What was the date you were referring to before?

Thompson: The first time we used lovastatin was in 1981 – the Alberts *et al.* paper describing it had just come out in 1980.[135] So that was pretty soon after. And I think nowadays plasma exchange is still regarded as the treatment of choice, and although we are not allowed to show slides at this meeting, I can't resist showing you a picture of one of the original homozygotes that we treated at the Hammersmith in the early 1970s; she is now in her mid-50s [died February 2006], and this shows her doing a fun run in Athens in May 2004, just before the last Olympics.

Bruckdorfer: It was suggested that I might talk a little bit about lipoprotein oxidation. The oxidation hypothesis in its infancy was against a background in which the discussion of antioxidants and free radicals brought a wry smile to many faces during the 1960s and 1970s, because there was quite a lot of conflict

---

[131] See Appendix 2, pages 85–6.

[132] Mevinolin was introduced by Merck & Co. in 1980 in the US and changed its name to lovastatin in 1986 [Alberts *et al.* (1980)]. For the background to Merck's development of this statin, see Vagelos and Galambos (2004): 132–63; Hawthorne (2003): 70–81, 90–2, 100, 105, 151–8, 243.

[133] Thompson *et al.* (1986).

[134] See, for example, Walker and Tobert (1987); Tobert (1987). Simvastatin became the first statin approved for over-the-counter sale by pharmacists for people at 'moderate' risk of a major coronary event. Royal Pharmaceutical Society, practice division (2004).

[135] Alberts *et al.* (1980).

about their significance to say the least, and even accusations of charlatanism in some cases. It was probably only the discovery of superoxide dismutase by Fridovich that brought it back into a sort of scientific acceptability.[136] But all of this really derived from the original discovery of Brown and Goldstein and the ensuing work, which was to do with how LDL actually bound to its receptor. And the approach was by Bob Mahley and others to modify lysine residues using diketene to acetoacetylate the LDL, and they found that that actually blocked the normal binding to the LDL receptor.[137] At the same time it was discovered that it also meant that this modified LDL would actually be taken up readily by the macrophage. I think that was a key discovery.

But, of course, this was just chemistry. The very important discovery by Fogelman, in Los Angeles at the University of California, Los Angeles (UCLA), is that if they modified the LDL with malondialdehyde, a product of oxidation, then the same thing happened.[138] Several people were working in this area; Anne [Soutar] started work on β-LDL I think at that time, with Brian Knight a year or two later. But the idea of the aldehyde was important, and attracted the attention of people such as Hermann Esterbauer.[139] Esterbauer was a chemist who had worked on aldehydes for years and was interested in them in biology, and realized that perhaps he could contribute to this in some way. Eventually, around about 1984, he discovered that if he modified LDL with another aldehyde, which was the major product of oxidation of fatty acids, essential fatty acids, 4-hydroxynonenal, that he could actually produce the same effect. Simultaneously, there was another strand of activity going on at San Diego in Steinberg's laboratory, where he found that you could actually modify lipoproteins simply by incubating them with endothelial cells or later smooth muscle cells.[140] It was realized, however, that probably they happened to choose a particular medium, Ham's F-10, which contains copper ions and ferric ions, which were helping to accelerate that process. In fact, the standard way in which oxidation was performed in the test tube was often by simply using these ions and not the cells. Nevertheless, they were able to show that this often led to uptake and formation of foam cells, and this became an exciting area and was

[136] McCord and Fridovich (1969).

[137] Weisgraber *et al.* (1978).

[138] Fogelman *et al.* (1980).

[139] Jurgens *et al.* (1986).

[140] Henriksen *et al.* (1981).

accepted. I picked that up at that particular time – Gus [Born] was talking about nitric oxide (NO) earlier, we didn't know NO was released by endothelial cells at that time, we all called it endothelium-derived relaxing factor (EDRF) – and found that oxidized LDL would inhibit the relaxation of blood vessels. At high levels of LDL, even nonoxidized LDL was also inhibitory but LDL was much more potent if it was actually oxidized. This ultimately led to the discovery of the scavenger receptor and its structure by Monty Krieger.[141] This led us almost to the position where we are now, to a greater understanding of gene expression induced by oxidized products. I think we just about get to the year 2000 level, the beginning of studies in which we find that vitamin E simply has no benefit as far as cardiovascular disease is concerned, leaving some to have egg on their faces on this particular issue. But, of course, they did all this work before they knew what the real oxidant was, and we still don't really know which oxidant actually caused the lipoprotein oxidation, nor whether or not vitamin E, and in particular vitamin C, would actually prevent oxidation *in vivo*.

Galton: Brown and Goldstein made their major discovery of lack of suppression of HMG-CoA reductase in fibroblasts of patients with FH. Now with the Hammersmith Hospital representatives at this meeting, Anne Soutar and Gil Thompson had patients with large families of FH, they were cultivating fibroblasts and I assume they knew how to measure HMG-CoA reductase in fibroblasts. Why didn't they make the same observations as Brown and Goldstein, since they were so well placed to do the experiments? What were you doing?

Soutar: I wasn't there. [Laughter] I was still in Houston working on lecithin: cholesterol acyltransferase (LCAT).

Thompson: I was in Houston too. [Laughter.] Brown and Goldstein were up the road in Dallas.

Oliver: I think we will solve that one at teatime.

Professor John Betteridge: We owe such a lot to this inborn error of metabolism, this experiment of nature called familial hypercholesterolaemia (FH). It led to the discovery of Brown and Goldstein's LDL receptor, etc., etc. Yet, it's interesting when you look back at how little influence it had on the acceptance of cholesterol as a risk factor of vascular disease. I remember when I first did lipid clinics with David Galton, seeing young men who had lost their brothers in their thirties. It really brought the cholesterol story home to me. I

---

[141] Krieger (1992).

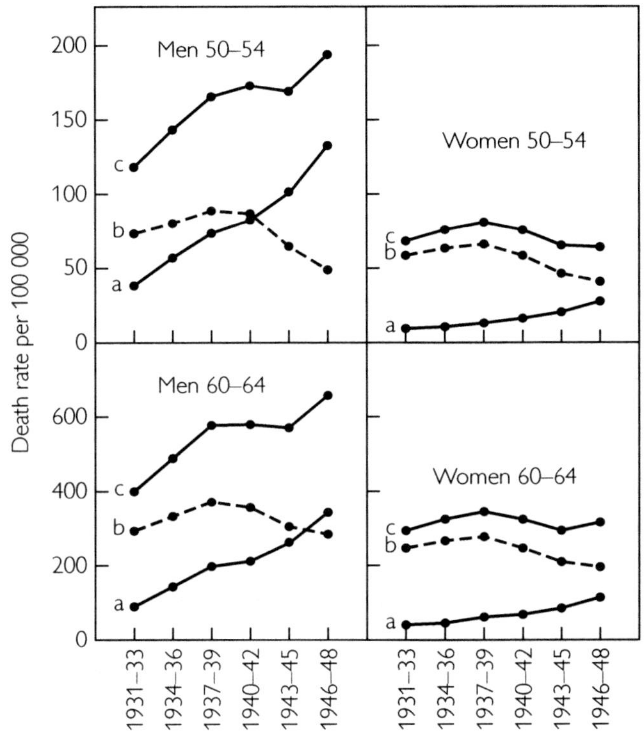

Figure 5: Mortality from heart diseases at ages of 50–54 and 60–64 in men and women, England and Wales, 1931–48.

a: diseases of coronary arteries, angina pectoris; b: chronic myocardial diseases, but including MI; c: sum of a and b.
Morris (1951): 1.

wonder why it didn't make a bigger impact. These were young men who were not smoking, who had normal blood pressure, yet they were dying early of heart disease. I think it's a paradox that it has helped all this research, but it didn't help the cholesterol story.

Oliver: We will move on to the next session and I am now going to ask the father of investigation in the UK, Jerry Morris, to open this session. We all know what Jerry has done and I hope that we can persuade him to talk a little bit about it, the London Hospital Survey and so on.[142]

Professor Jerry Morris: I will start with the London Hospital story in the 1950s. I come from social medicine, whose main method in investigation is *epidemiology*, but the emphasis is on *social* medicine.

[142] Morris (1951).

We were set up in 1948 by the Medical Research Council (MRC) as the Social Medicine Research Unit, essentially to investigate possible connections between people's health and the way they live.[143] We decided to deal with MI, a very serious disease, newly common, and which was apparently on the increase. In fact, when I was at UCH in the 1930s, the assumption then was that the disease was increasing [see Figure 5].

I will describe two early studies, published in detail in the *Lancet* in 1951 and 1953, both relevant to our concerns this afternoon.[144] The first probed the underlying pathology of the apparent alarming current increase of acute myocardial infarction (AMI). I analysed the post-mortem records at the London Hospital where the great Professor H M Turnbull had instituted routine description of the condition of the coronary arteries and the myocardium at *every* post mortem. Turnbull himself, Professor of Morbid Anatomy there, an extraordinary man, told me that he had learned when he was a postgraduate student in Professor Georg Schmorl's laboratory in Dresden, Germany, that in every post mortem you must record every abnormality you see, which Turnbull then proceeded to do.[145] I studied post mortems conducted on people in middle and early-old age between 1907–49, during the period that saw the emergence of AMI from obscurity to national and international priority. [See Table 1.]

The main findings can be summarized: first, coronary atherosclerosis was exceedingly common, near universal, throughout. Second, during those years there was a steep increase of fresh coronary thrombosis and associated AMI in both men and women. Finally, despite intensive search I was unable to find any indication of an increase of the underlying coronary atherosclerosis over those years; the indication indeed was of a decline.

Unfortunately, I was unable to replicate these observations. I could not find another teaching hospital *cum* pathology department where such routine recording was performed at post mortem, not in London or the provinces, nor Scotland, or even the Massachusetts General Hospital or Johns Hopkins. What was deficient everywhere else was the routine recording of the state of the coronary

[143] Dr J N (Jerry) Morris was Director of the Social Medicine Research Unit from 1948 until his official retirement in 1975, a member of the MRC staff and later a Professor at the London Hospital and the London School of Hygiene and Tropical Medicine (LSHTM). R M Titmuss was his colleague in the initial stages. The Unit was located at the Central Middlesex Hospital (1948–56), the London Hospital (1956–66) and the LSHTM (from 1966). See also Berridge *et al.* (eds) (2006): 33, 44, 56.

[144] Morris (1951); Morris *et al.* (1953)

[145] Turnbull (1915).

Years	Average number of necropsies per year at age of 35–70			
	Males		Females	Total
	Recent coronary thrombosis*	Acute myocardial infarction†	Both§	
1907–14	1.1	0.25	0.25	1.6
1915–18	2.25	0.5	0.75	3.5
1919–23	3.4	1.6	0.8	5.8
1927–31	3.6	1.2	1.4	6.2
1935–39	4.4	1.8	1.8	8.0
1944–49	5.5	3.0	2.0	10.5

Table 1: Deaths from coronary heart disease in the London Hospital, 1907–49.

* Fresh, unorganized thrombus, with or without acute infarction.

† Or necrosis or rupture; due to coronary atheroma; without recent thrombosis, though there was often evidence of *old* thrombosis.

§ Recent coronary thrombosis and/or acute myocardial infarction.

Excludes: cases of coronary embolism, occlusion by atheromatous debris and with syphilitic aortitis

Includes: cases with recognized diabetes; in 1907–14 there were 1 in 13 cases; in 1944–49 there were 7:3 in 53 men, and 4 in 12 women.

Adapted from Morris (1951).

arteries and myocardium in the great mass of noncoronary, nonvascular deaths from injuries, infections, cancers, that provided some indication of what was happening in the general population.[146] I gave up, much to the disappointment also of Harry Himsworth, the Secretary of the MRC, and in effect my boss, who had become deeply interested in these studies.[147]

Next, more straightforward epidemiology: we set up incidence studies of CHD among men in a wide range of occupations to give us information to go alongside the national mortality statistics. The studies included a huge range of occupations: medical practitioners, schoolteachers, factory workers and, very importantly, a range of occupations in London Transport and the civil service. In 1949 I had a hunch that AMI could be related to occupation. It was more common in men than women, in middle age than in youth, there were some hints in the national mortality data and Osler's ideas were often quoted, often by my own teacher in cardiology, the great Thomas Lewis.[148]

[146] Morris and Crawford (1958). Reports on a consecutive series of 25 necropsies in middle-aged males from an enquiry sent to all pathologists in Britain.

[147] Morris (1960).

[148] Osler (1910). See, for example, Lewis (1946). For the background to this period of clinical research in Britain, see Reynolds and Tansey (eds) (2000).

Within a year there was an intriguing suggestion of some protection against CHD, in particular against the most serious acute coronary syndrome – sudden death as first clinical manifestation – in the conductors of London's double-decker buses compared with the drivers, and in postmen *vs* three sedentary grades of office workers in government.[149]

We tested these observations in every way we could devise. We had arrived, quite unready, at the most difficult of situations, testing in effect a causal hypothesis without the possibility of experiment and dealing only with data that we couldn't manipulate.

Booth: May I just interrupt there. Sir John McMichael always told me that you went straightaway and showed your data to him at the Hammersmith. What did he say?

Morris: I will tell you privately what John said at tea![150]

Of equal importance to our agenda today, I must report the reception of these observations. There was a huge media response, with which I had no idea how to cope. More interesting was the response or, rather, the total lack of response, by the cardiology community. I register this only because of the striking contrast with the US. The Director of the National Institutes of Health (NIH), or rather, the NHI (National Heart, Lung and Blood Institute), flew over to see me for discussion of a follow-up. Paul White telephoned and we soon became friends, indeed, family friends. I well remember our first joyous dinner together, the four of us – at the Ritz, of course. More seriously, I hope that one of the outcomes of our deliberations today will be an assessment of the role of 'clinical science' in the national health and research effort, positive and negative.

I will conclude, personally, by reporting that we were soon struggling with the far more difficult issues of research into exercise in leisure time by a population rapidly becoming sedentary.[151] At the same time, we were adjusting to the new

---

[149] Morris *et al.* (1953).

[150] Professor Jerry Morris wrote: 'On Dr Himsworth's suggestion I showed Sir John McMichael our CHD findings on occupation and other population data we had been gathering, such as on ruptured heart. All illustrated that epidemiology, which some of us in England and the US were developing, could yield information different from and supplementary to the clinical and that from the lab experiment. He listened attentively, paused, then just said: "Rubbish". I departed. He came round, of course, in later years.' Note on draft transcript, 19 February 2006.

[151] See, for example, Morris *et al.* (1973, 1980); Chave *et al.* (1978).

world of 'risk factors' rapidly being established across the Atlantic. In brief, physical activity in time became recognized as some protection in the presence of one and of all of them.

Professor David Barker: In Jerry's unit was a young statistician called Martin Gardner, who moved down to Southampton. He decided to make a detailed map of the distribution of deaths from CHD in England and Wales over an 11-year period from 1968 to 1978. The map was the most detailed made, and it didn't discover anything new, but it did point up the paradox that CHD had its highest rates in the poorest parts of the country. There were two possible explanations for that: one is that people lived different lives, and were exposed to different diets and other influences in the areas with the highest rates, which were mostly in the north and west of the country; the other possibility was that the people in those areas were simply more vulnerable. It is not a new idea to think in terms of vulnerability. If you come to a place where there is a lot of tuberculosis, you immediately wonder: (a) are they being exposed to high doses of infection, or (b) are they more vulnerable to disease? At that time there were people interested in vulnerability to CHD, and Tony Mitchell was one. You will remember that Tony was Professor of Medicine in Nottingham and he once toured the country with his famous lecture: 'Should every cow carry a government health warning?'[152] He mused on the possible genetic vulnerability to CHD. If you think some people might be more vulnerable to CHD, then two questions arise: 'Is this vulnerability acquired through the chaotic processes of ageing, or is it acquired through the organized processes of development?' The latter would be a logical starting place. If you acquire vulnerability to CHD during development, at what point in development would that be? Here Martin's map was extremely helpful, because on his map London had a very low risk of CHD and that would point circumstantially to a link between resilience to heart disease and good intrauterine conditions. You could not possibly argue that it was good conditions in childhood because growing up in London in the early years of the last [twentieth] century, children were exposed to the conditions described by Charles Dickens. So Martin's map led to a hypothesis that good prenatal development is linked with resilience to CHD. The reason why prenatal growth in London was good was simply that London during the nineteenth century and early twentieth century, renewed itself constantly by bringing in some of the fittest young women from the southern and eastern

[152] See, for example, Mitchell (1984, 1985).

seaboard, where people were well nourished. The young women came into domestic service. Their babies had exceptionally low neonatal mortality.

The subsequent demonstration that people who had a low birth weight are at increased risk of CHD was received with some hostility.[153] Thanks to the excellent child health records in Finland we now know that children who later develop CHD grow differently, both prenatally, and postnatally.[154] They have slow prenatal growth; they have a period of two years' slow postnatal growth, thereafter they start to put on weight rapidly. They do not reach the average for other boys and girls until around ten. It's not the overweight child who is the problem, but the child who was underweight and then gains weight rapidly after the age of two. Hand in hand with the mounting epidemiological evidence has come an understanding of biological processes, which underlie the association between altered growth and CHD. For example, people who are six pounds rather than eight pounds at birth have fewer nephrons in their kidneys. We are beginning to understand how this may lead to hypertension, especially if it's attended by rapid weight gain and increased body mass index of childhood. We know that people who are small at birth set their metabolism in a frugal way, which may be inappropriate when in later life they are exposed to adequate or even excessive nutrition. We know that people who did not grow well in the uterus and were small or thin at birth are more vulnerable to the effects of low income in adult life, however that effect is mediated.[155] The field is coming on very fast, because an understanding of the process is now persuading those for whom epidemiology was no more than circumstantial evidence.

Oliver: Are there some questions before we move on about this particular subject? If not may I ask George Davey Smith please to take up the theme.

Professor George Davey Smith: I was asked to talk about what I was thinking about with regards to cholesterol from 1950 to 2000. As I was born in 1959, perhaps it was not very much. But I guess I will be one of the few people here who experienced the emergence of knowledge of this issue as a nonexpert. I can remember exactly where I was when I first heard about cholesterol: it was around 1971, I was walking in the Peak District and drinking a pint of milk in

---

[153] For example, Paneth and Susser (1995).

[154] For example, Barker and Osmond (1986); Barker *et al.* (1989); Barker *et al.* (2002); Kajantie *et al.* (2005).

[155] Barker (1972); Barker and Rose (1976).

every village, and the friend I was walking with said, 'This is going to give us fat on the heart, drinking these pints of milk'. So lower-middle class kids from Warrington harboured an opinion in 1971 and had heard about cholesterol, and I guess the knowledge was pretty widespread.

And indeed, the first work I did in this field, in 1985, was a survey of public attitudes about the causes of CHD, with 20 000-odd people in Wales being asked what they thought caused heart disease and two-thirds of them said saturated fat, high blood pressure and smoking.[156] When the same thing was done a few years later, even higher percentages chose them. So as far as the general public were concerned, I think there was reasonably widespread knowledge of at least what they were supposed to think caused CHD.

Talking about the epidemiology of cholesterol, by that stage large-scale pooling projects had been carried out, where all the big observational studies came together, and these had shown that there was a very strong consistent association between blood cholesterol levels and CHD.[157] I think that the first study done in Britain – but Jerry [Morris] might correct me here – was prospective by Ian Higgins and Archie Cochrane, who started measuring cholesterol in the Rhondda Fach studies in the late 1950s.[158] Then more prospective studies in Britain came out and the first major international pooling project appeared in 1978.[159]

The issue that I got involved with was one which I think became important in terms of thinking about strategies to deal with CHD, the observation in epidemiological studies that low cholesterol was associated with increased levels of mortality from causes other than CHD. This certainly became an aspect of the equation: what was the appropriate strategy for dealing with the positive association of cholesterol and heart disease? We carried out a study on brain cancer, my first prospective observational study, and showed a positive association of cholesterol with brain cancer.[160] One of my next papers was a study showing that there was no positive correlation in a different study, so it wasn't an auspicious start.[161] I was working on cholesterol and noncoronary

[156] Davey Smith and Nutbeam (1988).

[157] Pooling Project Research Group (1978).

[158] Higgins *et al.* (1963). See also Ness *et al.* (eds) (2002).

[159] Pooling Project Research Group (1978).

[160] Davey Smith and Shipley (1989).

[161] Davey Smith *et al.* (1992b).

mortality, and this was a popular issue since the apparent detrimental effects of low cholesterol had been reported in 1974 when the first major paper on low cholesterol predicting colon cancer had appeared.[162] The National Heart, Lung, and Blood Institute in the US organized a mass pooling project in the same way that had been done for CHD, bringing together all the major prospective studies to try to see if they could make any sense of these observations.[163] Geoffrey Rose and Michael Marmot were too busy to represent the first Whitehall study at this conference, so I was sent.[164] Our perspective came from looking at the Whitehall study, which was different from many of the other studies, as it had data on social factors: civil service employment grade (which was very strongly predictive of CHD mortality, and mortality from other causes), data on marital status, and data on health status and respiratory function. We showed that if you didn't take all these things into account then it did, indeed, appear that people with low cholesterol did badly with respect to a whole range of noncoronary causes of death. If you took into account all those confounding factors, however, then it appeared that these were noncausal associations, the association between low cholesterol and non-CHD mortality being due to the confounding factors and to the fact that being ill, or having conditions that led to poor lung function also led to low cholesterol.[165] Other reports came out regarding this association, however. But the early cholesterol-lowering trials with drugs – although not diet – also suggested an increase in the risk of non-CHD mortality, which we proposed might be due to effects of the drugs then in use to lower cholesterol,

---

[162] Rose *et al.* (1974).

[163] Pooling Project Research Group (1978).

[164] The first Whitehall study in 1967 involved 17 718 men, aged from 40–64 years, in the British civil service. Men in the lowest employment grades were more likely to die from CHD and other causes than those in the highest grades. After controlling for standard risk factors it was found that those in the lowest grade still had a relative risk of 2.1 for CHD compared with those in the higher employment grades. In 1985 the Whitehall II study was set up to determine the underlying causes for these differences, and included women. All non-industrial civil servants, aged 35–55 years, in the London offices of 20 civil service departments were invited to take part in a cardiovascular screening examination at their workplace. Of those invited, 10 308 (73 per cent) participated in the baseline survey. In addition to the screening, the participants were given a self-completion questionnaire. From the initial survey it was found that employment grade was associated with work control and job demand with lack of control related to long periods of absence. Since its inception there have been a further six phases of the Whitehall II study, the most recent completed in September 2004. See www.phis.org.uk/doc.pl?file=pdf/Heart%20Health%20Practice-primary%20prevention.doc (visited 2 November 2005).

[165] Davey Smith *et al.* (1992a).

not to low cholesterol itself.[166] This effect has not been seen in the statin trials. In the end, the trials resolved that issue, rather than the observational studies. We thought we demonstrated to our satisfaction that there was no causal link between low cholesterol and noncoronary causes of death, but it wasn't to everyone's satisfaction.[167]

I would like to finish by agreeing with John Betteridge's point about the lack of strength that people put on the observation of genetic hyperlipidaemias. Looking back now with respect to cholesterol and non-CHD mortality, there's a letter by Martijn Katan in the *Lancet* in 1986, which pointed out that it's very difficult to identify causal effects in observational studies. People who get sick end up with low cholesterol and people who smoke have low cholesterol levels, and these would lead low cholesterol levels to be related to increased mortality. However, Katan argued that being sick doesn't change your genotype and your genotype is unrelated to smoking and all the other confounding factors. Therefore, if low cholesterol was causally related to increased risk of colon cancer, people whose genotype was associated with lower cholesterol levels should have an increased risk of colon cancer.[168] I can remember reading Martijn Katan's *Lancet* letter at the time and thinking, 'This is nonsense', but now I think that the concept it advanced is probably one of the most important additions to observational epidemiology in the past half century.[169]

Barker: The first time I spoke to the American Heart Association meeting I had a remarkably small audience. I said to the organizer that considering there were 15 000 cardiologists attending the meeting, remarkably few were in the room. 'What am I competing with?' He replied that there was a lecture in the next hall on income tax for cardiologists.

Pyörälä: As you said, David, cardiologists showed very little interest in the results of epidemiological studies. It was, however, interesting that with the publication of the first angiographic trials on the effect of lipid-lowering on the progression of coronary atherosclerosis, their attitudes to the cholesterol issue began to change, perhaps because these studies were carried out using their own

---

[166] Principal Investigators (1984); Davey Smith and Pekkanen (1992b).

[167] Davey Smith *et al.* (1992a, 1993); Davey Smith and Pekkanen (1992b).

[168] Katan (1986).

[169] Keavney (2004); Davey Smith and Ebrahim (2003).

tools.[170] One reason why repeated observations from epidemiological studies on a continuous relationship between serum cholesterol and CHD extending over the whole cholesterol distribution did not ring any bells in the minds of cardiologists and other clinicians, may have been the way of expressing 'normal' values for biochemical measurements as ±2 standard deviations around the mean in healthy subjects. Thus, even very high cholesterol levels were within the 'normal range'.

Oliver: In no way would I even think of defending cardiologists, since they were the source of much inertia for a long time. Why is this? Having run two cardiac departments, I think the answer is two-fold: the first is that most cardiologists are not academically trained. I am not even sure how inquisitive they are. Second, they are very busy pushing tubes into patients. I can remember when I was in Sweden, Lars Carlson came up with the phrase: 'Of course, cardiologists are two-parameter men, aren't they? Not three-parameter men.' By two parameters, he meant flow and pressure. I had a lot of people in my team doing cardiac catheterization, but they did not think much about the causes of coronary disease.

Scott: I don't think we can blame the cardiologists for what was happening in the early 1980s. There was huge resistance in the popular press to the idea that diet and cholesterol might really cause CHD. That might have come from the cardiologists, but I think it was more general. I think that maybe we in Britain are offshore islanders, who are not going to be told what to do! It wasn't until the big statin trials that this view was reversed.[171]

Tunstall-Pedoe: This is getting into the area that I am going to talk about after tea, but I think British academic medicine had as much to answer for as cardiologists in terms of resistance to coronary disease prevention.

Professor John S Yudkin: Is it not a resistance to this diet–cholesterol–heart hypothesis that we are talking about, rather than resistance to the cholesterol hypothesis? I agree with John Betteridge that until the 1980s we had no effective pharmacological tools to lower cholesterol. The diet studies were all on polyunsaturated fatty acids, which were all a little bit iffy, as they may have had other effects on the heart independently. So I think conflating diet and heart and cholesterol was probably where the problems lay.

---

[170] Brensike *et al.* (1984); Blankenhorn *et al.* (1987); Brown *et al.* (1990).

[171] Scandinavian Simvastatin Survival Study (4S) (1994).

Oliver: I think that's right and I don't think that the World Health Organization clofibrate trial helped – for which I was responsible and to which I will make reference later – it added to the uncertainty because of its largely negative findings. Cardiologists and many internal medicine physicians rather rubbed their hands and said, 'I told you so.'

Booth: May I just interject with a point, because it's probably an interesting fact of modern history that the word fibre has not been mentioned.

Oliver: Tom Sanders is going to talk about diet later.

Betteridge: I remember when I first started seeing patients with what was called 'maturity onset' diabetes in the early 1970s, the main focus was on glucose. Blood lipids were not routinely measured. Even other important risk factors, such as blood pressure and cigarette smoking, were not addressed.

I remember being taught that the disease in the arteries of people with diabetes was somehow different from the atheromatous disease in people without diabetes. It seemed to me at the time that it was accepted that people with diabetes would die of heart disease and stroke, and there was nothing that could be done about it.

In terms of research in lipids and diabetes there was a focus on adipose tissue, lipolysis and free fatty acids and David Galton was at the forefront of this in the UK.[172] It is of interest that this area of research has come full circle and currently is a hot topic in relation to the Metabolic Syndrome.

I remember that there was interest in plasma triglycerides and vascular risk in diabetes, and the name of Dr M J Albrink in the US comes to mind.[173] Of course, the importance of low HDL as a vascular risk factor was 'rediscovered' by Miller and Miller in their *Lancet* paper in the 1970s.[174] They referred to the early work of David Barr in the US in the 1950s and subsequently Esko Nikkilä in Finland. Professor Nikkilä also highlighted the low HDL levels in diabetes.[175]

---

[172] Clifton-Bligh and Galton (1976); Reckless and Galton (1980).

[173] Albrink and Man (1958); Albrink *et al.* (1963); Albrink (1964).

[174] Miller and Miller (1975).

[175] Barr and Russ (1951); Nikkilä and Hormila (1978).

Lipid and lipoprotein turnover studies were in their infancy, but increased hepatic lipoprotein synthesis was described in diabetes, together with decreased clearance due to reduced activity of lipoprotein lipase.[176] Around this time new, more simple techniques were becoming available for the measurement of individual lipoproteins and the calculation of LDL by the Friedewald formula.[177] In addition, the measurement of cholesterol (and triglyceride) became easier with the development of enzyme assays. In this regard, the name of Dr Bill Richmond, consultant clinical chemist at St Mary's, deserves mention as contributing to the development of the assay for cholesterol.[178] This, of course, liberated laboratories from all the acid needed for the Lieberman–Burchard reagent;[179] Dr John Reckless, Professor David Galton and I contributed one of the first cross-sectional studies relating the presence of symptomatic concentrations in diabetic people, published in the *British Medical Journal.*[180]

The idea of qualitative changes was emerging. Some of the early studies with electrophoresis suggested that some patients with diabetes had the broad beta band suggestive of remnant particle accumulation. Then, of course, the LDL subfractions described by Ron Kraus appeared.[181] I think it was the US Multiple Risk Factor Intervention Trial (MRFIT) screenees study that showed us the risk of cardiovascular disease in diabetes in relation to cholesterol, very important in the mid-1980s.[182] People with diabetes with a low cholesterol level had a risk two to three times higher than a nondiabetic person with a high cholesterol level. I think that's very important and the US Framingham Study contributed to that.[183] Then there was the issue of clustering of multiple risk factors and everyone claims this as their own as far as I can see. It was put on the map by

---

[176] Oliver and Boyd (1953b).

[177] See Glossary, pages 141–2.

[178] Richmond (1973, 1974, 1976).

[179] Robertson and Cramp (1970). This required a substantial amount of concentrated sulphuric acid.

[180] Reckless *et al.* (1978).

[181] Austin *et al.* (1988, 1990).

[182] Multiple Risk Factor Intervention Trial (MRFIT) (1976).

[183] The Framingham Heart Study started in 1948 with a sample of 5209 men and women aged from 30–62 years in Framingham, Massachusetts, US, and was directed by the National Heart Institute. The subjects have returned every two years for further tests and 5124 children of the original sample were recruited in 1971. Gordon *et al.* (1977). See www.nhlbi.nih.gov/about/framingham (visited 18 November 2005).

Gerald Reaven's 1988 Banting Lecture, but you know Markold Hanefeld in Dresden published on it in 1981, and Crepaldi earlier.[184] We have all seen this associated risk factor clinically, but I think it was Reaven who put that together, and, of course, acknowledged Himsworth, of whom we have heard already, who was one of the first to point to the difference in diabetes, the insulin-resistant diabetes, compared with the insulin-deficient diabetes.[185] Then, of course, the relationship of clustering of risk factors to insulin resistance, which may be the central abnormality, was identified and, I think, an important player was Edwin Bierman in Seattle.[186] Another thing that came out of Finland was the idea that the dyslipidaemia is present when diabetes is diagnosed, and that again suggested a phase before diabetes, where you have dyslipidaemia developing. Now, of course, we talk about Metabolic Syndrome pre-diabetes and that's where the focus of attention is.[187]

I was taken by Elliot Joslin, the diabetes physician and my hero in diabetes, who in 1927 said something that I thought was fantastic.[188] He asked if it was possible, chemically, that the high prevalence of atherosclerosis in diabetic patients could be attributed to the high-fat diets patients had received and particularly those rich in cholesterol? He thought this was the case and was determined to keep the cholesterol in the blood of his patients at a normal level. He suggested that this therapeutic procedure be open to experimental investigation and that it should not take long to solve. He said that in 1927. When I first talked about cholesterol in diabetes, my colleagues attacked me because people with diabetes had enough to contend with. Cheese was freely available on the diet, carbohydrates were restricted, but cheese with saturated fat was free and patients could eat as much as they liked.

Galton: I agree with everything that John Betteridge said, because after all I taught him most of it! [Laughter.]

Betteridge: He taught me *all* he knew. [Laughter.]

Yudkin: If we are concentrating on the cholesterol–heart hypothesis, I said earlier that I think where a lot of doubt existed was the belief that the cholesterol–heart

---

[184] Crepaldi (1971); Julius *et al.* (1981); Reaven (1988); UK Prospective Diabetes Study (UKPDS) (1991).

[185] Himsworth (1936).

[186] New *et al.* (1963).

[187] Laakso (1995).

[188] Joslin (1927). See also Joslin (1956).

hypothesis would be exactly the same paradigm as the diet–heart hypothesis.[189] I think they mean two different things: cholesterol being only one of the mechanisms whereby diet can influence CHD. But I suspect that I am not the only person to continue to see patients who ask, 'How can I have a high cholesterol? I hardly eat any fatty foods, animal foods, drink any milk?' Or my diabetic patients who say, 'My sugar can't be high, because I haven't had any carbohydrates.' There is that misunderstanding.

I think the other is something where I would agree with John Betteridge, that there has been a growing recognition of the multiplicity of risk factors that cluster together, especially in people with diabetes. But you don't need diabetes to have all the diabetic risk factors. So the classic diabetic dyslipidaemia of the high triglyceride, low HDL, the microalbuminuria, central obesity, the high plasminogen activator inhibitor type 1 (PAI-1) levels, a whole range of things that are almost universally linked with type 2 diabetes, are pretty common indeed in the 25–50 per cent of the UK, and 98 per cent of the population of the US, with obesity, as a Metabolic Syndrome.[190] I think there is something about obesity that ties these together, superimposed on what is a little switch in the blood glucose, which makes you diabetic. But as John said, that probably doesn't make that much difference to cardiovascular risk.

I think that the one thing that we haven't considered or haven't mentioned anywhere this afternoon, is the growing field of low grade inflammation with C-reactive protein as a marker – whether this is completely independent of the cholesterol–heart link or whether it ties in somehow, perhaps in terms of LDL oxidation, or some other effect on scavenger receptor uptake. My belief is that there is a link between adipose tissue composition and low-grade inflammation, which underlies links between these various things that cluster together as the insulin resistance syndrome and I think that that is completely independent of the cholesterol–heart link. My view is that lipids are important in diabetes, but different lipids. The whole of the recognition of risk in Metabolic Syndrome is a separate construct from the diet–cholesterol–heart relationship. It complements it, but comes from a completely different direction and the two factors together may well have some bearing on the diet–heart paradigm. Chairman, you quoted from John French at the beginning of the meeting, that in CHD there are changes in the vessel wall on the one hand, and prothrombotic changes on the

---

[189] For a view of butter and the diet–heart link in New Zealand, see Steel (2005).

[190] Yudkin J S (1993, 2000); Foyle *et al.* (1995); Yudkin *et al.* (Caerphilly Study) (2002).

other hand. It may well be that these inflammatory things are more to do with the plaque complication, its rupture or thrombosis, while the cholesterol may be more to do with vessel wall damage.

Professor Paul Durrington: I think that John [Betteridge] did a very nice summary and I entirely agree with everything he said. I must say I have some reservations about this multiplicity thing when it comes to coronary disease. I fully recognize that in a society like Britain coronary disease clearly has a number of different risk factors. However, cholesterol is pre-eminent and is the permissive factor allowing other risk factors to operate. I think one of the things that we have not really covered today is the transnational epidemiology of CHD. Something that greatly disturbs me is that those nations where coronary disease is really still rare, are beginning to acquire a higher rate of coronary disease, and the big thing that is happening there is a nutritional change leading to a rise in their cholesterol. In most countries where there is coronary disease, by and large the middle-aged male population has cholesterol of more than 4mmol/l.[191] Fat, particularly saturated, comprises a high proportion of dietary energy and obesity is common. In those countries where coronary disease is uncommon, they derive most of their dietary energy from carbohydrate and obesity is uncommon. Yet we know that in China and India, all that is changing and they are very populous countries. We are actually on the verge of a pandemic of coronary disease far greater than we have ever seen before. We think we are beating it here, and we are, but coronary disease is not due to deficiency of statins. It is also not, by and large, a deficiency of genes; it is nutritional. I think that was why people had a lot of trouble accepting the cholesterol hypothesis in Britain. When all we could do to lower cholesterol was to criticize the food and agricultural industries, and to talk about diets, there were great forces ranged against people who wanted to lower cholesterol. These industries killed a lot of the enthusiasm for nutritional change by their promotion of negative views. I don't want to talk about individuals, but it was very obvious that if you had certain speakers at a medical meeting their lectures would be organized and arranged by the food industry. In the early days of gene work as well, the suggestion that coronary disease was genetic was publicized because it was a distraction from nutrition. When statins came along then we had a big industrial force raised behind cholesterol-lowering with drugs. Statins have undoubtedly been a great boon. They have been a great success and we haven't yet seen their full benefits, but we shouldn't lose sight of the fact that one casualty of statins has actually

---

[191] See Glossary, pages 139–40, for a comparison of US and European measures of cholesterol. See also note 198.

been the nutritional hypothesis. For most parts of the world where coronary disease is going to be important in the future, it is a nutritional problem. It can only be tackled nutritionally: drugs are too expensive there. I think that point has been lost sight of and it worries me greatly.

Oliver: In view of the subject of the meeting, were you thinking that way 25 years ago?

Durrington: I didn't have much choice then, Michael. We had no very effective cholesterol-lowering drugs. I was always very impressed by the differences between different nations in their coronary rates: rural Africa, South America, Asia as I have mentioned, and Britain. It seemed to be a message that we weren't taking up and we should have done then and still need to do now.

Born: It's a very good discussion. I wonder whether it's permissible to draw brief attention to an experimental contribution to the aetiology of diabetes? Professor Yarom and her colleagues in Israel showed that when rats are made diabetic with streptozotocin, the density of negative electric charges on arterial endothelium is reduced within a month by about a third – very significant indeed.[192] So on the basis of our evidence presented earlier that this charge slows the movement of LDL into arterial walls, I think that there is very likely a causative connection between these experimental observations and the well-established fact that the clinical manifestations of atherosclerosis occur earlier in diabetics.

Scott: Our own interest in the Metabolic Syndrome of insulin resistance has increased progressively over the past several years. This was initially driven by the recognition that we were going to get on top of cholesterol as a risk factor, and that obesity was driving the Metabolic Syndrome of insulin resistance and all of its serious downstream consequences (including proatherogenic lipoproteins, high blood pressure, hypercoagulation, type 2 diabetes, atherosclerosis) and was emerging as the dominant risk factor. Thus I echo and re-emphasize everything that John [Betteridge] said.

Oliver: I think we will move on from this session. I should say that this morning I had a telephone call from Gerry Shaper who said that he had been tying his shoelaces and got an extreme pain in his back and couldn't possibly move. I asked him what he was doing, and he replied, 'Can't you hear, I am sitting in a chair groaning?' That's his apology because he was scheduled to speak at this point.[193]

---

[192] Raz *et al.* (1998).

[193] See Appendix 2, pages 85–6.

Tunstall-Pedoe: I am pleased to be here. I have two problems. One is that I haven't made any earth-shattering discoveries myself. I have just tried to find how to put things into perspective and perhaps to help others as well, by doing so.

The second is that I tend to like people I disagree with more than those who agree with me. I intend to upset everyone who is here and if there's anyone who's left out, I apologize. What I would like to do is to set the medical–cultural scene in coronary disease and cholesterol when I got into coronary disease epidemiology in the late 1960s and subsequently.

Dr Wallace Brigden, my consultant cardiologist boss at the London Hospital, took me to visit Professor Jerry Morris at the London School of Hygiene and Tropical Medicine (LSHTM) in 1969 to talk about Jerry's proposal to recruit someone to set up a heart attack register in the London Borough of Tower Hamlets in east London. At that time I was training as a cardiologist and in general medicine. I was a registrar hoping for promotion to senior registrar, but had been told to do some research first.

Like other hospital doctors in training and medical students at that time, I knew exactly where coronary disease came from. It came out of ambulances and disappeared about three weeks later, leaving a box of chocolates behind it if it had survived. Hospital doctors had nothing to do with angina. Angina was dealt with by GPs; hospital doctors dealt with acute emergencies, rather than chronic diseases, which were rather undignified and also were more properly dealt with by GPs. I was a bit puzzled when I started working with Jerry Morris to discover that coronary disease was officially classified by epidemiologists as a chronic disease, because I had only seen acute medical emergencies. Dr Wallace Brigden warned me on the way to the meeting that epidemiology was not considered quite respectable by many cardiologists, particularly those at the Hammersmith. By implication such research might be considered a waste of my first-class Cambridge degree and I should really be going into a laboratory. To be fair he did not press this argument too hard or say he agreed with it, but he thought I ought to know.

Epidemiology also was equated with drains, rather disparagingly. The other thing at that time that respectable doctors were not into was prevention. A doctor was concerned, traditionally, with diagnosis and treatment and anything else was snake-oil salesmanship. If you were an academic, you were not supposed to be enthusiastic about preventing disease. It was a bit like an accusation under the Joseph McCarthy era [1940s–50s] in the US that those of doubtful politics had been prematurely antifascist; if you were in favour of prevention you were unbalanced, lacking in judgment and an object of deep suspicion. What was needed was more and more research.

The burning academic argument at that time was that if you didn't know all the causes of a disease, you couldn't do anything about it, and it had the convenient logical consequence that it was never the right time to do anything about the disease, but always right to call for more research. Of course, that was utter nonsense, but it was based on a false concept of disease causation that risk factors were additive, so tackling one alone was tinkering at the edges, rather than a multiplicative model, where if you can affect one risk factor in a big way you can have a major effect on disease rates, which is what prevention is about, now belatedly substantiated by the effect of statins.

Going back to when Winston Churchill was Prime Minister in the 1940s, it was said that the British Cabinet was divideded between 'war-wagers', or 'better-notters'.[194] I think you could classify most medical academics in the 1960s and 1970s as 'better-notters'; there were always arguments why you shouldn't do anything about coronary disease and why you couldn't prevent it. At the top of the ivory tower of academia, were the lipodologists. They existed only in major teaching hospitals in large centres of population, collecting extremely rare conditions. They lived in a sort of Alice-in-Wonderland world confusing the very big and the very small; the very rare and the very common. If you read a chapter on cholesterol by lipidologists there would be a photograph of a patient with bizarre skin and joint lesions caused by FH, which was allegedly responsible for the most common cause of death, CHD, killing one person in three. Most photographs would be of the same patient, because they were so rare. You were supposed to be looking out for him or her in the outpatient clinic, but they never turned up. Meanwhile epidemiologically raised cholesterol levels were so common they were classified as 'normal range'.

Cholesterol was something that Americans had; it definitely wasn't British. Anyone who talked about cholesterol was obviously suffering from American-style hypochrondria. If a patient asked what they should do to stop themselves from getting coronary disease, it was evidence that they were mentally unbalanced. No fit person, it was thought, should worry about becoming ill.

As for measurement, only a fool would measure cholesterol, because you couldn't smell it, you couldn't taste it, it didn't hurt you, and also you couldn't measure it

[194] Gilbert (1991).

at all reliably. If you measured it twice in the same patient, you got two different answers. When I was studying people from South Asia in my coronary register in Tower Hamlets I produced the original results showing that they had an excess of coronary disease over the cockney natives, I was puzzled by why the two branches of the London Hospital seemed to have different cholesterol levels.[195] I split samples between them and they were 20 per cent higher in Mile End than in Whitechapel, enough to be of enormous significance epidemiologically. When I asked the physicians about it, they said they knew. The two chemical pathologists concerned both insisted that they were getting it right and the other one was wrong. But for that I might have done a pioneering study of risk factors in British Asians, as it was I could not trust the results.[196]

The other thing about risk factors – remembering that this was the era when there was an argument about whether blood pressure was a mixture of two populations or whether it was continuously distributed[197] – was that clinicians divided things into normal and abnormal. If it was normal, you could go away and forget about it; if it was abnormal, then it justified the enormous indignities and treatments piled upon you. This was an era when normal was a diastolic blood pressure of 104mmHg – sorry I mentioned blood pressure – and normal cholesterol was below 300mg/dl (7.8mmol/l).[198] There was no point in measuring it if most people had normal cholesterol anyway.

An epidemiologist should not be quoting case histories, but just very briefly. Three patients and the presence or absence of cholesterol readings: one I saw in the London Hospital medical unit's outpatients' clinic. There was a young woman who had been put on a most ferocious diet as the result of a high cholesterol reading (over 300mg/dl). I didn't believe that she could have got her cholesterol down to just over 200mg/dl on this diet in one go, and had great difficulty in persuading her to come off it for three months so I could see whether the original reading was right. She had been put on this ferocious diet,

---

[195] Tunstall-Pedoe *et al.* (1975); Tunstall-Pedoe (1975, 1978).

[196] Professor Hugh Tunstall-Pedoe wrote: 'Cholesterol standardization came later, after similar problems were experienced in the clofibrate studies, which involved Michael Oliver and Jerry Morris and his unit.' Note on draft transcript, 8 January 2006.

[197] Swales (ed.) (1985).

[198] Cholesterol readings are expressed in two ways: the European Système Internationale (SI) unit (one millimole is a value expressed per litre as mmol/l and gives information about the concentration of a solution) and the US expression mg/dl [milligram per decilitre]. See Glossary for normal cholesterol levels, pages 139–40.

which meant that she couldn't eat with anyone else, or ever eat out, on the basis of one cholesterol reading. When I took her off the diet, the cholesterol was only slightly higher, but it was perfectly satisfactory. The original reading was wrong and had never been replicated.

I saw a man in the Tower Hamlets heart attack register that I did with Jerry Morris.[199] Well, I didn't see him, but I interviewed his widow. He had had an attack of chest pain in the night and the emergency doctor had come along and said that it was indigestion, and nothing to worry about, and he died before morning, his wife finding him dead, downstairs on the sofa at daylight. He had been admitted three years earlier to St Bartholomew's Hospital and I noticed on his notes that his cholesterol had not been measured when he had his MI or afterwards. The interesting thing was that he was only 28 years old when it first happened, but it was not considered necessary in 1968 to measure the cholesterol levels in a young man with a coronary in a London teaching hospital.

Later in the 1970s at St Mary's Hospital, London, among the patients referred for various reasons I saw an airline pilot in his forties whose cholesterol had been measured in a research project. It was over 300mg/dl and the team referring him wanted to take him off flying completely and planned to do some coronary angiograms. His other risk factors were normal, apart from his cholesterol, and he ran three miles every day, with no family history. There was this idea that cholesterol levels over 300mg/dl were terrible, and that nothing need be done when the levels were under 300mg/dl.

Then there was diet. The Seven Countries Study complemented the US Framingham Heart Study and showed a good triangular relationship between diet, cholesterol levels and coronary disease.[200] The treatment for elevated cholesterol in those days, apart from some perfectly disgusting drugs that have now been replaced, was to give people a diet sheet. When they came back nothing much had happened unless you got regression to the mean from the initially high readings. Failure to respond to diet sheets created a myth of a diet-resistant type of hypercholesterolaemia. It was not the cholesterol resisting the diet, but the patient resisting the diet sheet.

As has been pointed out, there was an enormous amount of negative propaganda going on, which, to me, is of as much historical interest as the discoveries that challenged it. We see progress as papers published in prestigious journals and

[199] Tunstall-Pedoe (1978).

[200] Keys (1970).

'miracles of modern medicine', but the negative propaganda going on through the 1970s and 1980s in give-away medical magazines and brochures was quite incredible.[201] Much of this was directly or indirectly sponsored by vested interests that sought out mischievous mavericks, who would be given equal or greater prominence than everybody else. Even respectable medical journals like the *BMJ* and the *Lancet* liked to publish comments and articles from mischievous mavericks. [Lots of laughter] Even as late as 1993, I can remember attending a meeting that I had organized with Douglas Chamberlain, then President of the British Cardiac Society, on risk factors for cardiologists. This was when secondary prevention wasn't well established, and cardiologists were thoroughly suspicious of the term 'prevention' anyway. The meeting was told by an eminent cardiologist from a teaching hospital not too far from here (outside London), that the *BMJ* had proved that cardiologists could forget about cholesterol. That was 1993, just before the results from the Scandinavian 4S study came out.[202] Since then cardiologists have not been allowed to forget cholesterol, but 90 per cent of the evidence was there already. It was not just cardiologists, but academic medicine which had inertia and resistance as well. I rest my case there.

Oliver: Can I make a comment there, substantiating what you were saying. I don't think that it was really recognized by the majority of cardiologists that cholesterol needed to be measured until about 1980, maybe a bit before. This was not a routine in Britain and as you rightly say if you did it you were a suspect American.

Tunstall-Pedoe: There was also the argument that after you had had your coronary heart attack, your cholesterol was irrelevant to your prognosis. That was an argument that went on until very recently, and it is wrong. The same applies to other major risk factors after MI.

Booth: I was taught my biochemistry in the University of Dundee, then the University of St Andrews, and the biochemist who taught me in the 1940s was R P Cook, the man who wrote the Cook book.[203] I have no doubt whatever that

---

[201] See Butter Information Council pamphlet, '*The Search': A film review of research and diet and coronary heart disease. Notes and summary script* (undated). Among the specialists appearing in the film, presented by Dr Tom Margerison, was Dr Elspeth Smith. A copy of this pamphlet, provided by Professor Hugh Tunstall-Pedoe, will be deposited along with other records of the meeting in Archives and Manuscripts, Wellcome Library, London.

[202] Scandinavian Simvastatin Survival Study (4S) (1994).

[203] Cook (ed.) (1958).

my memory is absolutely correct in saying that cholesterol was thrust down our throats, and furthermore he used to wave the corpses of rabbits that had been fed cholesterol at us and their blood vessels were stained a vivid red, I can remember it to this day. Obviously R P Cook should not be forgotten. Three cheers for R P Cook.

Oliver: He's not been forgotten. I actually mentioned him in the introduction.[204] He wrote his book in 1958, which was on the physiology and biochemistry of cholesterol and that as far as I know was the first book in this country on the subject of cholesterol.

Marks: I think one of the reasons why cardiologists thought cholesterol had nothing to do with them was because normally they would only have their patients' cholesterol measured immediately or soon after the patient arrived at hospital following a MI, when, of course, it was low. Some of us tried to suggest that they might repeat the measurement when the patient had recovered completely; but this was seldom done. It is a fact, scarcely recognized at the time, that plasma cholesterol – or more properly, lipoprotein – levels go up and down, just like any other acute phase proteins in response to injury. That's why cardiologists couldn't see the association, because their patients never had high plasma cholesterol levels at the time it was measured.

Oliver: Of course in the cardiological literature even as late as the early 1980s, certainly in the 1960s and 1970s, there was very little about cholesterol and nothing about lipoproteins. The *Journal of Lipid Research*, or the *Journal of Clinical Investigation*, were the main fora, but that sort of journal was too erudite for most cardiologists to read.

Davey Smith: Briefly on this point, observational studies had established that high blood cholesterol levels caused CHD by the 1970s. The trials which we are going on to talk about, caused concern about the effects of lowering cholesterol on noncoronary mortality. All the meta-analyses of trials showed that cholesterol reduction was associated with reduced CHD, so the issue wasn't so much whether cholesterol was a risk factor for CHD. The question was whether the methods available for lowering cholesterol, which includes some of the drugs that have been mentioned (that is, fibrates and resins), were producing benefits? And that was the issue, I think, not whether cholesterol was a strong causal factor for CHD. I think from most epidemiological perspectives, as Paul Durrington was saying, the very strong determinancy of cholesterol with respect to population differences

[204] See note 24.

in CHD was clear and recognized. However, some population differences could not be attributed to cholesterol. There's Paul McKeigue's very important work on CHD among people with Indian heritage, who as a group had lower cholesterol levels than a group of European-origin people, and who had very high levels of CHD despite this.[205] If you looked in the Whitehall Study, at the large social class differences in CHD, there was a four-fold difference in CHD risk between the lowest grade of civil servants (high) and the administrators (low). However, the administrators had higher cholesterol levels than the lower-grade civil servants.[206] Similarly in the studies that Victor Hawthorne started in Scotland in 1964, there were big social class differences in CHD, and there were social class differences in cholesterol.[207] The problem was the social class gradient in cholesterol ran in the opposite direction to the social class differences in CHD.[208] Cholesterol levels were higher in people who could afford more meat. The third population difference which, I think, is important here was the very sudden emergence of a big gender difference in CHD in Britain. In Jerry Morris' book, *Uses of Epidemiology*, the first edition of which appeared in 1957, it is clear that the CHD epidemic was largely seen in men, a finding confirmed in later editions of the issue.[209] Now the coronary epidemic was an epidemic in men and there's no evidence of a sudden emergence of a cholesterol difference between men and women. So there were some population differences that couldn't be explained by cholesterol. But I think the general agreement would now be that cholesterol was the most important risk factor concerning population differences, but it did not account for all population differences.

Oliver: It would be incorrect if I didn't mention Geoffrey Rose, whom we haven't mentioned in the entire meeting yet.[210] He was the leader in cardiovascular epidemiology in the UK in the late 1960s and the 1970s. Many will have read his book and his papers, and I just want to place on record that Geoffrey Rose was an architect of great importance in this field.[211]

---

[205] McKeigue *et al.* (1985).

[206] Marmot *et al.* (1978).

[207] Hawthorne *et al.* (1969); Furst *et al.* (1972); Hawthorne (1977); Hart *et al.* (1999).

[208] Davey Smith *et al.* (1997).

[209] Morris (1957); Lawlor *et al.* (2001).

[210] See notes 103 and 162.

[211] Rose (1981).

Professor Thomas Sanders: I want to comment on a few key papers, particularly George and Norman Miller's paper in the *Lancet*, which really drew attention to low levels of high density lipoprotein cholesterol (HDL) as a risk factor and its relationship to insulin resistance or the Metabolic Syndrome, particularly in the Asian population.[212] I think it started a different way in which we looked at blood cholesterol and paved the way to look at the fractions that carried cholesterol.

Until that time it was believed that the higher the blood cholesterol, the greater the risk. It is worth recording that Barry Lewis' research on LDL synthesis and metabolism clearly showed that the higher the level of LDL cholesterol, the greater the severity of disease (atherosclerosis), and that this was driven by the rate of very low density lipoprotein cholesterol (VLDL) synthesis and the rate of LDL catabolism. What emerged from the Millers' paper was that low levels of HDL cholesterol were a more powerful, predictive factor than total or LDL cholesterol. The paradox of the lower risk of cardiovascular diseases in females in spite of their higher levels of blood cholesterol (at least post-menopause) could, in part, be explained by this. There was also discordance between men and women in the pattern of changes in risk of CHD in the postwar period: it is interesting to note that the rates of CHD fell in women from about 1956 while they were rising in men.[213] One of the potential explanations for this may have been a change in oestrogen-related diseases, which were actually rising at the same time, such as breast and ovarian cancers. It is well known that serum oestradiol levels increase with increasing body fat levels, particularly in post-menopausal women. We now know that oestradiol helps keep total blood cholesterol levels low by increasing LDL receptor numbers, but at the same time it increases HDL cholesterol, which is protective. I suspect many of the changes in blood cholesterol initially attributed to diet can be explained by hormonal effects.[214]

---

[212] Miller and Miller (1975).

[213] DHSS, Committee on Medical Aspects of Food Policy (COMA) (1984). Professor Philip Randle, Chairman. See also Randle *et al.* (1990). Professor Tom Sanders wrote: 'The 1984 COMA report was the first report that advocated changes in dietary fat composition and followed on from the Royal College of Physicians Report in 1976. Professor Tony Mitchell dissented from the main recommendation to decrease saturated and total fat. Although he is not named, it is stated: "The tenth member believes that this evidence is insufficient but that benefit may accrue insofar as the recommended change in diet contributes to the avoidance of obesity." Section 4.1.11.' E-mail to Mrs Lois Reynolds, 7 March 2006. See also Truswell (1984).

[214] Grundy (1991).

Scott: I have listened with interest to what George Davey Smith has said, and think that the Metabolic Syndrome of insulin resistance emerges as two to three times more prevalent and a dominant risk factor in the absence of smoking. I don't know about prevalence in women, but smoking is an issue for them too. Diet is of poor quality in those with low income and those that are economically deprived, a common feature in the past in parts of north-west Britain and in many of the large cities. This contrasts with the much better diet of those who are better off, such as those in the civil service. If one looks at the British national food survey[215] then the real difference between north-western cities such as Glasgow and Belfast is not in the amount of cholesterol and saturated fat consumed in these cities relative to London, but rather in the small quantity of fresh fruit and vegetables, and grain in the diet.

Oliver: Well, it still applies doesn't it?

Scott: Yes.

Thompson: I would like to comment briefly on Hugh Tunstall-Pedoe's broad spectrum criticism of virtually everybody in the place. I wasn't quite sure which he thought was the bigger crime: lipidologists measuring cholesterol, or cardiologists not measuring it. But as far as the dismissive attitude of the latter towards the diet–cholesterol hypothesis goes, I entirely agree with you. One of my colleagues at the Hammersmith, not Sir John McMichael, used to say a cholesterol-lowering diet won't make you live longer, it will just make life seem longer.

Tunstall-Pedoe: If I could just comment further on lipidologists. The problem was that lipidologists made things extremely complicated with systems of classification. Any document on coronary prevention produced for other doctors was dominated by lipidologists from lipid clinics, was about 80 pages long and virtually unreadable, through all the subclassifications it had. No two of these ever agreed with each other, but you were expected to know and understand them or you weren't safe treating cholesterol. You were expected to defer to

---

[215] The Dietary and Nutritional Survey of British Adults, 1986–87 was a one-off cross-sectional survey of 2197 individuals aged 16–64 living in private households in Great Britain, undertaken by the Social Survey Division of the Office of Population Censuses and Surveys (OPCS) and the Ministry of Agriculture, Fisheries and Food (MAFF). The National Diet and Nutrition Survey programme (NDNS) was established in 1992 by MAFF and the Departments of Health to provide a comprehensive cross-sectional picture of the dietary habits and nutritional status of the population of Great Britain, to be repeated every eight to ten years. For an overview of health benefits of physical activity in 2001, see www.parliament.uk/post/pn162.pdf (visited 12 January 2006).

the specialists, but there was no way that the tertiary specialist clinics in major teaching hospitals were going to be able to tackle the causes of coronary disease in the whole population.

I think it's a problem. I am being really provocative now. If you are a high priest to a mystery, you don't want to simplify things, because if there's no need for complexity, you don't need any high priests.

Booth: I am very sorry that Gerry Shaper is not here to present his own position.[216] I remember meeting Gerry in Kampala, Uganda, in the early 1960s when Denis Burkitt, his colleague, was doing his work on the lymphoma that bears his name. Gerry found a tribe in northern Kenya called the Samburu and they were an interesting tribe, because they chased a herd of cattle all day, and lived on milk, so they had an extremely high milk diet, and a cholesterol intake well above normal. The argument, I believe, was that they ran 40 miles a day, chasing their cattle. If anybody can corroborate that statement, I would be grateful.[217]

Durrington: I was only going to point out that there is a gene variant proprotein convertase subtilisin/kexin type 9 (*PCSK9*), which has only recently been described in people from the African continent and causes low cholesterol.[218] Some of those tribes that you referred to, I suspect, may have a gene that stops them having high cholesterol. For example, their women during pregnancy don't have a rise in cholesterol either. This is a fascinating area. Years ago it was used as evidence that a high fat diet did not cause coronary disease. I think what this does illustrate, therefore, is one of the problems that we had in this field, which George Davey Smith also has highlighted. Although the bulk of the evidence is blindly pointing us in one direction; people argue by finding small minutiae and odd things that don't quite fit with the main part of the evidence, and somehow their views have become prominent. I think that is a problem that we have had over the years.

One other thing: this business about gender difference, which again was big during the period that we have been discussing, this belief that oestrogen protects us against coronary disease.[219] I am pleased to see that we are now learning from

[216] See Professor Shaper's brief comments in Appendix 1, pages 81–4.

[217] Shaper (1962).

[218] Cohen *et al.* (2005).

[219] Oliver and Boyd (1953a); Boyd and Oliver (1956).

the error in this. It is not oestrogen that protects against coronary disease, it's androgens which predispose to it. That's what all the clinical trial evidence tells us.[220] If you look at the gender difference in coronary risk it is the amount of HDL in women compared with men that seems best to explain their different risk. Boys and girls have very similar lipids until puberty, and it's at puberty in the boys that the HDL drops and then remains lower throughout life.[221] It is not that the women have oestrogen to protect them, it's that men have androgens that predisposes them to coronary disease.[222] There was a dominant belief that somehow oestrogen and femininity were protective against coronary disease in the period that we are talking about. Now randomized controlled clinical trials have shown that this is not the case.

Oliver: We are going to move on now to the final session about drugs and diet developments and I am going to ask Tom Sanders to talk about diet.

Sanders: In order to understand the main drivers for changes in food production it is worth considering the backdrop of postwar Britain when there were food shortages and rationing. A major aim was to attain self-sufficiency in food from Britain and to develop modern technologies to produce substitutes for existing natural products that depended upon imports. That the National Institute of Research in Dairying at Shinfield in Reading employed over 200 scientists underscores the commitment to improving the production of milk and milk products. Unilever Research and Development at Colworth House, Bedford, had major research programmes focusing on producing cocoabutter substitutes.[223] Some of the technologies developed facilitated lipid research, in particular the invention of gas–liquid chromatography and its application to analysing lipids by Tony James at Unilever and Archer Martin at NIMR, who received a Nobel Prize for his earlier work on liquid–liquid chromatography.[224]

---

[220] Hulley *et al.* (1998); Writing Group for the Women's Health Initiative Investigators. (2002); Grady *et al.* for the HERS Research Group (2002).

[221] Christensen *et al.* (1980); Rifkind and Segal (1983).

[222] Durrington (2003).

[223] For early background of the National Institute for Research in Dairying, see Kay (1951); for Unilever work, see, for example, Padley and Timms (1978). Unilever holds a 1960 patent, GB827172, covering their early work on cocoabutter substitutes.

[224] Archer Martin and Anthony T James developed gas–liquid (partition) chromatography (GLC) in 1950. He and James used the new column to separate a variety of natural products, which he announced in his Nobel Prize lecture in 1952. See James and Martin (1954, 1956); Martin and James (1956).

An odd ball, Hugh Sinclair wrote an extremely long letter entitled 'Deficiency of essential fatty acids and atherosclerosis et cetera', published in the *Lancet* in 1956, where he expounded the view that atherosclerosis was related to a deficiency of essential fatty acids and he proposed that the hydrogenation of fats produced trans-fatty acids that caused essential fatty acid deficiency.[225] Sinclair proposed that atherosclerosis was due to a deficiency primarily of linoleic acid. It was a rambling letter that touched on many facets. Kinsell and Sinclair later expounded the view that the essential fatty acid content of dietary fat was the primary factor responsible for lowering blood cholesterol. In this paper he clearly refers to linoleic acid as being the 'essential fatty acid'.[226] Hugh Sinclair in later times referred back to that original *Lancet* letter with different interpretations, particularly to suggest that CHD was due to a deficiency of n-3 fatty acids. He appeared to embellish his story as he went along. However, this idea that the type of fat, rather than the total amount of fat in the diet, matters stimulated a lot of controversy and research on the relationship between the type of fat and blood cholesterol.

The work in the South African group, led by Bronte-Stewart, showed that fish oil, which did not contain linoleic acid but was rich in long-chain polyunsaturated fatty acids of the n-3 series, lowered blood cholesterol.[227] In the 1960s and the 1970s, outside the UK, there was a lot of research going on by Ancel Keys, Francisco Grande and Mark Hegsted, who came up with predictive equations for the effects of saturated fatty acids, 12 to 16 carbon atoms long, on blood cholesterol, and the lowering effect of polyunsaturated fatty acids.[228] Monounsaturates were seen to be neutral. In the UK the Keys view was rejected as being involved in type of fat, or level of fat. You need to appreciate the backdrop in the UK and the view that butter, cheese – dairy

---

[225] Sinclair (1956). See also Ewin (2001); Sanders (2001).

[226] Kinsell and Sinclair (1957).

[227] Bronte-Stewart *et al.* (1956).

[228] Professor Tom Sanders wrote: 'The Keys predictive equations are: Δ plasma cholesterol = $(2.3\Delta S\text{-}\Delta P)$ + SQRT(Δ dietary cholesterol/1000kcal) Δ plasma cholesterol where ΔS is the change in energy provided by saturated fatty acids and ΔP is the change in energy provided by polyunsaturated fatty acids. These equations have been modified by Mensink and Katan [(1992)] who have estimated the effects of different fatty acids on LDL and HDL cholesterol. These showed that the equations of Keys tended to overestimate the effect of saturated fatty acids on LDL cholesterol.' E-mail to Mrs Lois Reynolds, 7 March 2006. Keys *et al.* (1957); Hegsted (1959).

products – were presented as being healthy food.[229] The view that these foods may be linked to increased risk of heart disease was seen as an attack on British farming achievements as well as eating habits and were ridiculed by several eminent researchers, such as Professor Tony Mitchell at Nottingham and Sir John McMichael at the Hammersmith.[230] Professor John Yudkin, the uncle of the John Yudkin here, had argued that there had been no change in fat intake in the postwar period when the epidemic of CHD had occurred.[231] He said the main dietary change was an increase in sugar, not dietary fat. He pointed the finger at sugar, which he later referred to as 'pure, white and deadly'.[232] He argued that hyperinsulinaemia induced by high intakes of sugar was responsible for the epidemic of cardiovascular disease. His views on sugar were not accepted because they did not affect total cholesterol levels.

In the early 1970s, Jim Mann's group at Oxford, Stewart Truswell and David Jenkins in London reported on the cholesterol-lowering effects of dietary fibre. They showed that some forms of dietary fibre, particularly the soluble type, lowered blood cholesterol. At that time I worked with Frey Ellis at Kingston Hospital, London, and we were able to show that strict vegetarians (vegans) had astonishingly lower serum cholesterol concentrations, about two-thirds of the values seen in the general population.[233] The argument turned on how much of this was due to a low dietary saturated fatty acid intake, lack of cholesterol, lower body weight and also ingestion of dietary fibre and plant proteins, such as that provided by soy. Our own data suggest that most of the difference could be explained in terms of saturated fatty acid and cholesterol intakes. It is now quite well established that if you put people on these extreme sorts of diet, you can achieve very big reductions in serum cholesterol, equivalent to those achieved with drugs such as statins.[234] The real problem is that it is difficult to get people to conform to such diets in the long term.

---

[229] See note 201.

[230] McMichael (1979); Mitchell (1985). Professor Tom Sanders wrote: 'Sir John McMichael aggressively attacked the lipid hypothesis. At the time it was widely alleged that he acted as a consultant for dairy interests.' E-mail to Mrs Lois Reynolds, 7 March 2006.

[231] Yudkin (1964).

[232] Yudkin (1972).

[233] Professor Tom Sanders wrote: 'David Jenkins, Stewart Truswell and Jim Mann [Simpson *et al.* (1981); Mann *et al.* (2001); Venn and Mann (2004)] showed that soluble fibre lowered plasma cholesterol, but that cereal fibre such as wheat fibre did not have this property.' E-mail to Mrs Lois Reynolds, 7 March 2006. Sanders *et al.* (1978).

[234] Jenkins *et al.* (2005).

The other driver in this has been the food industry, which developed modified products to lower blood cholesterol. Unilever developed a margarine rich in linoleic acid that was called 'Becel', short for blood cholesterol-lowering margarine, but they weren't allowed to call it that here in the UK and introduced it as *Flora* in the UK in 1965.[235] There were all sorts of implied claims put on the label – low in cholesterol, free from cholesterol, high in polyunsaturates or pictures of an electrocardiogram on the package or a logo of one of the heart charities – and this engendered a lot of confusion between dietary cholesterol and blood cholesterol in the mind of the public and among health professionals.[236] Foods containing cholesterol, such as eggs and shellfish, were labelled as potentially bad and people started to get the idea that cholesterol was bad for you, and that there was a direct link between dietary cholesterol and blood cholesterol. There had been work in the US, but not so much here, showing that cholesterol in large amounts increased blood cholesterol. Jim Mann's work in Oxford showed that it made very little difference whether you ate three eggs a week or six eggs a week.[237] This added to the public's confusion regarding diet and blood cholesterol. In retrospect, perhaps there was too much expected from the replacement of butter with margarine. Indeed, work by researchers at Unilever published in the 1990s showed that the substitution of 25g of polyunsaturated margarine for 25g of butter only lowered total cholesterol by 2.6 per cent and LDL cholesterol by 4 per cent.[238] So although there was abundant evidence that modifying the intake of saturated fatty acids and cholesterol could lower blood cholesterol, in practice it was difficult to achieve reduction greater than 5 per cent in blood cholesterol by replacing high fat dairy products with low fat varieties and using polyunsaturated margarine in place of butter.[239] However, this is hardly surprising if the impact of the relatively minor dietary changes are compared with the various predictive equations.[240] Peter Elwood's work in

---

[235] Unilever Health Institute [Vlaardingen, The Netherlands] developed Becel at the request of Dutch physicians for a margarine rich in linoleic acid and low in saturated fatty acids. Launched in 1960 it was sold at pharmacies in a can. For further background details, see Upritchard *et al.* (2005). See also the history of Unilever's involvement with margarine at www.unilever.com/ourvalues/sciandtech/How_where/ufhri/our_history/ (visited 12 January 2006).

[236] Sanders (1987, 1988).

[237] Edington *et al.* (1989).

[238] Hendriks *et al.* (1999).

[239] Tang *et al.* (1998).

[240] Sanders (1988).

the Caerphilly heart disease study showed that very little (about 5 per cent) of the variation between individuals in blood cholesterol levels could be explained by variations in the intakes of saturated fatty acid or cholesterol.[241] A finding later confirmed in the Dietary and Nutritional Survey of Adults in 1988.[242] We now recognize that cholesterol, particularly LDL cholesterol, increases with age independently of changes in the fat composition of the diet, which may be due to a decline in thyroid activity as well as changes in oestradiol levels in women following the menopause. Insulin resistance, which is associated with central obesity, increases LDL levels and lowers HDL cholesterol. These and other factors seem to explain much more of the variance in blood cholesterol within the UK population than differences in saturated fatty acid and cholesterol intakes.

Returning to the point made by Paul Durrington, that between-country studies, such as the Seven Countries Study, show that two-thirds of the variation in median cholesterol level appear to be explained by the difference in saturated fats intake and cholesterol intake.[243] In the southern Mediterranean diet 70 per cent of fat comes from olive oil, which is low in saturated fatty acids, and they eat little fatty meat and dairy produce. The changes that we are seeing in many developing countries, which tends towards a northern European diet high in animal fat, are accompanied by an increase in blood cholesterol.

Oliver: Now if anybody wants to add their experiences with diet.

Tunstall-Pedoe: I will mention the Masai. If Gerry Shaper was here he would say that one of the points about these people in these areas is that they are on the verge of malnutrition for a large part of the year while being very active physically. Therefore trying to extrapolate from them to a sedentary population is a mistake.[244] But the Masai and the Inuit were produced as the jokers in the pack by the food industry and the resistance movement of 'better-notters' until very recently. When my daughter went to an interview for entrance to Oxford University some years ago she was asked about risk factors, because of me, and

---

[241] Fehily *et al.* (1994). See also Ness *et al.* (eds) (2002): 79–82, 86, 127–9; Reynolds and Tansey (eds) (2005): 81–4.

[242] For background of the survey, which confirmed the lack of a strong relationship with saturated fatty acid intake and cholesterol, see note 215.

[243] Keys (1970); Keys *et al.* (1984).

[244] See Appendix 1, pages 81–4.

gave an orthodox account. The response was: 'What about the Masai? (giggle, giggle, giggle)'. I think the answer is: 'Well, what about the Masai?' That's the end of the argument. But the Masai and the Inuit were quoted right through to the end of the 1990s as the wild cards that showed that nothing could or should be done about coronary disease, and 'we need more research', right up until the statin trials came out. Now they appear marginalized and you do not hear about them any more, although they remain of theoretical interest.

Oliver: I think I should make an unprepared comment about Hugh Sinclair. I was at one of the Magdalen College meetings of the Atherosclerosis Discussion Group and Hugh asked me to stay in his house, Elspeth [Smith] was there too, and we had a rather late night, and the next morning we were given eggs and bacon. Hugh had some filthy stuff that he was drinking, which he said was tea. Well, it wasn't tea, it was seal oil. Elspeth – never short of a remark or two – in the kitchen, which was piled with filthy dishes because Hugh lived alone, asked, 'What is that? What is in the fridge, Hugh?' And Hugh was forced, very reluctantly, to find a key. Having spotted an ice pick hanging by the side of the fridge, Elspeth and Hugh opened it and inside was a frozen seal, at which he had been picking away. So he turned himself into a seal over a period of about three months.

The story doesn't quite finish there, because one day when I was doing something unimportant at home, the telephone went and it was Hugh saying, 'I want to have a liver biopsy tomorrow for fatty acid analysis. A doctor in Oxford doesn't think it is very wise. He said my bleeding time is 60 minutes. Is that high?' I replied, 'Well, you do what you like, Hugh, but it will be the last time you will be talking to me, or anybody else for that matter.' He didn't have it.

Hollman: Just a very quick clip on diet which you may not have read in the *New Scientist*.[245] Pekka Puska, born in Vaasa, northern Finland, in 1945, was director of the North Karelia Project in eastern Finland from 1972 to 1997.[246] He related a story of an elderly man from a small village near the Russian border who spoke to him after his talk: 'Doctor, you have spent a long time telling us what kind of fat we should put on our bread, but you haven't asked us what we do use.' 'Oh,' said Puska, 'What do you put on your bread?' Answer: bear's fat [very saturated fat].

---

[245] Neroth (2005).

[246] Puska *et al.* (1981).

Barker: To remind you about the origin of margarine.[247] Margarine was first used by the French army for lubricating pistols. Then Napoleon III advertised a competition in order to get more fat into the peasants' diet, but he didn't want them to eat anything as expensive as butter. Somebody cleaning his pistol with margarine thought, 'Why don't we submit this for the competition?' It won, and that is how we got margarine.[248]

Scott: I have to say that the explorer Sir Ernest Henry Shackleton is one of my heroes. He had tremendous survival skills in bringing his shipwrecked crew to safety after two years of privation on the southern polar ice. It is a story full of irony. Some of the crew, after their rescue, were rapidly sent to the front in the First World War, where they died. Shackleton himself died in 1922 at the age of 48 of a massive coronary on his journey back to the southern ice, while making a stop at the island of St Georgia. This may not have been helped by his diet of penguin and seal meat in the absence of any fruit and vegetables, but the most notable thing about Shackleton is that he always had a cigarette in the photographs.

Pyörälä: May I mention that the late Professor Geoffrey Rose, a famous lecturer in epidemiology, used to say that even small changes in lifestyles, when taken up in the population, may result in large benefits. My friend, Arthur Hollman, has told the story of North Karelia in Finland. We had the world record, not only in CHD mortality, but also in the population mean for cholesterol, almost 7 mmol/l, in the beginning of the 1970s. Now our population mean-cholesterol levels are down to 5.5 and CHD mortality has gone down by more than 70 per cent in men and women. Calculations done some time ago have shown that about 50 per cent of that decline is due to the change in the distribution of cholesterol, which is explained by dietary changes.

Sanders: May I briefly comment on the Finnish North Karelia study. It is often cited as a demonstration that a population approach to modifying fat intake is effective in reducing the average blood cholesterol concentration. One very big confounding factor in Norway and Finland was the consumption of boiled coffee, which is found to have a very potent hypercholesterolaemic effect and changes in the type of coffee preparations may also be a factor in that study.[249]

---

[247] For a cultural history of margarine, see van Stuyvenberg (1969).

[248] Fernandez-Armesto (2001).

[249] Aro *et al.* (1987); Pietinen *et al.* (1990).

Pyörälä: This has been taken into account in the published statistics.

Betteridge: I just wanted to say that we haven't really mentioned functional foods, which raised hackles among dieticians. My own view is that we have something that actually works, is acceptable and lowers LDL cholesterol. The evidence is good for the stanol esters and plant sterols incorporated into spreads and other products.[250] Of course they give extra benefit in patients on statins. I think those are interesting developments. They raised a lot of issues because they are expensive, but I think they are useful.

Oliver: We will move on to drugs. In 1956, George Boyd and I embarked on the first clinical trial in the UK of the effects of lowering plasma cholesterol in patients with CHD.[251] It was a fairly disastrous pilot study that would never have been permitted now. We recruited 100 male patients and gave 200μg ethinyl oestradiol (a large dose) to 50 and lactose to the other 50. All the treated men developed gynaecomastia. After five years, total cholesterol had fallen in the oestrogen-treated group by 18 per cent and was unchanged in the control group. But there was no difference in coronary morbidity and mortality between the groups. We concluded in 1961 on this minimal evidence that reduction of serum lipids after MI did not improve prognosis.

The first cholesterol-lowering drug to be tested in the UK was chlorophenoxyisobutyrate (CPIB), which was initially called *Atromid*® or *Atromid-S*® and later was named clofibrate. The story behind this is interesting.

In 1954, ICI had developed phenyl ethyl acetic acid as an insecticide. When sprayed from the air over fields near Clermont-Ferrand, France, many farm workers became ill and were admitted to hospital. Jean Cottet, the physician there, found that their blood cholesterol levels were extraordinarily low.[252] A chemist working in ICI at Macclesfield, Jeff Thorp, recognized the potential of this substance and later synthesized the analogue, chlorophenoxyisobutyrate or CPIB.[253] He approached George Boyd and me, and for three years we studied its effect on plasma cholesterol and lipoproteins in animals. In the early 1960s,

---

[250] Law (2000).

[251] Oliver and Boyd (1961).

[252] Cottet *et al.* (1954).

[253] Thorp and Waring (1962).

we reported its lipid-lowering effect in man.[254] As a result, several fibrates were developed and continue to be used particularly for treatment of mixed hyperlipidaemia. Chris Packard will take up the theme later. We weren't able to measure triglycerides in those days. The fibrates are much more effective, as we now know, on triglyceride levels. That led us into the WHO clofibrate trial, in which a key person was, of course, Jerry Morris. When it turned out that we could actually lower cholesterol using clofibrate – I am talking about 1964 – I took myself off to the Central Middlesex Hospital, where Jerry was working to discuss what we might do about it. And he brought in Austin Heady as our statistician, and to cut the story short, in 1978 we published the results.[255] The comparisons were between the two high cholesterol groups, each with 5000 otherwise healthy men.

The clofibrate trial was the first primary prevention trial. It was conducted in Edinburgh, Prague and Budapest and recruited 15 700 men. There were 5 300 in each of two hypercholesterolaemic groups – one received 2g clofibrate daily and the other identical capsules containing 400mg olive oil. There were two control groups, a high cholesterol and a low cholesterol group, [three groups in all]. There was a 9 per cent reduction in total cholesterol, a significant 20 per cent reduction in nonfatal MI but no decrease in fatal events. There was, however, a significant increase in noncardiovascular mortality. This was not specific but caused much concern. There was also an increase in the incidence of gallstones.

These results were encouraging but worrying, leading to the question as to whether reduction of raised plasma cholesterol would lead to a trade-off, as it were, between less MI and an increase in noncardiovascular mortality. Indeed, these results from the biggest primary prevention trial at that time (the 1970s) acted as a brake against intervention for another 16 years when the results of the first statin trial, the 4S study, were published.[256]

There were other drugs: MER 29 and triparanol. I hope that Chris Packard will say a word or two about them. I think it would be true to say that from about 1978 to the results of the 4S trial in 1994, there was a limited enthusiasm for trying to lower cholesterol, and that was largely due to the anomalous and still unexplained result of the WHO clofibrate trial.

---

[254] Oliver (1962a and b).

[255] Principal Investigators (1978).

[256] Scandinavian Simvastatin Survival Study (4S) (1994); Strandberg *et al.* (2004).

Professor Stuart Pocock: Not a British trial, but you could just, remember cholestyramine in the Lipid Research Clinics (LRC) trial, which is an example of over-placed enthusiasm I think possibly, because they were showing reductions in protein lipids, but very borderline significance for the actual reduction of coronary deaths.[257] And that's the trial I saw more of as a sales pitch than any other trial that I have seen. Cholestyramine was not a great idea, was it?

Packard: I think it is worth spending a moment on the intellectual landscape at the time. When the Lipid Research Clinics (LRC) trial came out, there was heavy promotion of cholesterol lowering.[258] American cardiologists and lipidologists became aggressive interventionist communities, whereas the British were more reserved. This is, perhaps, a noble interpretation. Certainly we were being dubious of the full benefits of cholesterol lowering and wanted more data than the LRC trial provided.

The other thing that was important at the time was the picture that we had of the progress of coronary disease, that is the growth from small lesions to big lesions that eventually blocked the artery. What mattered, we believed, was how to make the lesion smaller, and so produce clinical benefit. To go back to what Professor Woolf was saying earlier, that paradigm shifts are the key. Between the time of publication of the LRC trial and the first statin trials there was a major paradigm shift in the field of atherosclerosis. We began to understand that it was the fragility, not the size, of a plaque that mattered.[259] When we put together the protocol for the West of Scotland Coronary Prevention Study (WOSCOPS) trial we borrowed heavily from the Helsinki Heart Study trial, because it was very well done.[260] We also knew we were going to have to persuade the great and the good in the UK, and so decided to have some sceptical people on our team, and there was no one better than yourself, Chairman [Michael Oliver], having had the experience of the clofibrate trial. We were testing the benefits of primary prevention, because we knew that the 4S trial, a secondary prevention trial, was underway, the CARE and LIPID studies were being done at the same time by Squibb [Bristol-Myers Squibb], the company that marketed the statin, *Pravachol®*

[257] Brensike *et al.* (1984).

[258] The Lipid Research Clinics (LRC) Coronary Primary Prevention Trial was a National Heart, Lung and Blood Institute (NHLBI) primary prevention trial using the drug cholestyramine. See LRC (1984). For further details of the trial, see www.clinicaltrials.gov/ct/show/NCT00000488 (visited 24 January 2006). See also Table 2, page 76.

[259] Davies (1996).

[260] Frick *et al.* (1987); WOSCOPS Study Group (1995); Shepherd *et al.* (1995). See also Table 2, page 76.

(pravastatin sodium),[261] and we felt that primary prevention was the single biggest question that would need to be answered between 1995 and 2000. The onus was on us, not only to prove benefit, but also that cholesterol lowering carried a low level of risk. The need to do this was emphasized by bad press, just after we started.[262] The intellectual climate now became one in which people were looking for the benefit-to-risk ratio, recognizing that the drugs had risks associated with their use. That mood continues to the present day. We are still trying to find what benefit-to-risk ratio is acceptable if we intervene to produce very low cholesterol levels. In 1995 we all sat in the University of Glasgow halls and heard the results, and we were surprised at how good they were. The trial showed that statin use gave a third risk reduction in CHD and, against all predictions, a reduction in total mortality, although the P values were the most cruel that one could observe at $P = 0.051$: a P value of 0.049 is significant, while 0.051 is not. If we adjusted for risk factors, total mortality was reduced, with a P value of 0.039. So there was a 20 per cent reduction in mortality.[263] [See Table 2.]

These results helped change the landscape for coronary prevention and made it on to the front pages of most newspapers in the Western world. What was important for medicine was that the mood had changed. The 4S trial was the big watershed for cardiologists and WOSCOPS was a strong addition to that. One of the most remarkable things that came out of the trial when we examined the data carefully was that there was no lag period before benefit began. In the LRC and Helsinki nonstatin studies, there was a period of about two years before benefit began, and that was in line with the idea that regression of the lesion in size was critical.[264] Ours was the first trial to show clearly the benefits started within months of starting therapy, and those who saw the data unblinded early on found that it started from almost day 0. It is what I call a true 'intention to treat' analysis, as soon as you 'intended to treat' the person got the benefit. The reduction in risk continued as a straight line for the next five years. What is going on? Either the reduction in LDL is so powerful that you get benefit straightaway with stabilization of plaque, or the pleotropic effects of the statin start acting immediately; that is, the drug causes plaque stabilization directly within months of starting therapy. So WOSCOPS was a landmark trial like 4S.

---

[261] Sacks *et al.* (1992); Prospective Pravastatin Pooling (PPP) project (1995); LIPID (Long-Term Intervention with Pravastatin in Ischemic Disease) Study (1995).

[262] Davey Smith and Pekkanen (1992a).

[263] WOSCOPS Study Group (1997).

[264] Lipid Research Clinics (LRC) Coronary Primary Prevention Trial (1984); Frick *et al.* (1987).

Trial	Drug, diet or intervention	Patients	Reference
Oslo diet–heart study (1970)	changes in diet: low saturated fats; low cholesterol; high polyunsaturated fats	412 M; 30–64 yrs; post MI; 11 yr follow-up; Norway	*Circulation* (1970) **42:** 935–42.
WHO clofibrate study (1978)	clofibrate	10 627 M; hypercholesterolaemia; 30–59 yrs; free of CHD; 5.4 yr follow-up; UK	*British Heart Journal* (1978) **40:** 1069–118; *Lancet* (1984) **ii:** 600–04.
Lipid Research Clinics (LRC) study (1984)	cholestyramine resin; fat-restricted diet	3806 M; 35–59 yrs; Type II hyperlipoproteinaemia; free from CHD; USA	*Journal of the American Medical Association* (1984) **251:** 351–64; 365–74.
Helsinki heart study (1987)	gemfibrozil 600mg twice daily	4081 M; 40–55 yrs; dyslipidaemia; primary-prevention trial; Finland	*New England Journal of Medicine* (1987) **317:** 1237–45.
DART (1989)	changes in dietary fat, fish, and fibre intakes	2033 M; <70 yrs; post MI; 2 yr follow-up, UK	*Lancet* (1989) **ii:** 757–61.
POSCH (1990)	partial ileal bypass	838 M + F patients; post MI hypercholesterolaemia; 7 yr follow-up; USA	*New England Journal of Medicine* (1990) **323:** 946–55.
4S (1994)	simvastatin 20–40mg	4444 patients, 81% M; mean age 60; angina or previous MI; cholesterol 5.5–8.0mmol/L; 5.4 yr follow-up; Scandanavia	*Lancet* (1994) **344:** 1383–9.
WOSCOPS (1995)	pravastatin 20–40mg	6 595 M; 45–64 yrs; elevated LDL; UK	*New England Journal of Medicine* (1995) **333:** 1301–7.
CARE (1996)	pravastatin 40mg	3583 M and 576 F; 21–75 yrs; previous MI; elevated LDL; USA	*New England Journal of Medicine* (1996) **335:** 1001–9.
LIPID (1998)	pravastatin 40mg	9 014 M + F; 31–75 yrs; previous AMI or unstable angina; Australia	*New England Journal of Medicine* (1998) **339:** 1349–57.

Table 2: Double-blind randomized controlled trials before 2000.[265]

[265] Leren (1970); Principal Investigators (1978); Lipid Research Clinics (LRC) Coronary Primary Prevention Trial (1984); Frick *et al.* (1987); Burr *et al.* (1989); Buchwald *et al.* (1990); Scandinavian Simvastatin Survival Study (4S) (1994); Shepherd *et al.* (1995); Sacks *et al.* (1996); Long-Term Intervention with Pravastatin in Ischemic Disease (LIPID) Study Group (1998).

It changed medical practice, and, I think, it changed our thinking about what was possible with cholesterol lowering.

Oliver: On a point of history: when was the WOSCOPS trial conceived?

Packard: It was conceived in about five minutes in 1988. I was away when my colleague Jim Shepherd went to a meeting at the Glasgow Western Infirmary and the story goes as follows. A senior director from the sponsoring company, Squibb, was visiting Scotland, his home country. He got together with the local cardiologists and asked for suggestions for prevention studies. The cardiologists said they wanted to do a secondary intervention trial, which Squibb was planning elsewhere. As this director was putting on his coat to leave, Jim said, 'Wait a minute, we want to do a primary prevention trial.' Jim had worked on the LRC trial, a primary prevention trial in Houston, Texas, and I had been there with him. We were invited to submit a protocol and within a few days we sent it by courier. The rest is history. I think Squibb deserves a lot of praise because it went looking worldwide for ideas and groups to do this sort of thing. This was long before the publication of the 4S trial.

Oliver: Stuart, you were the statistician and a very important part you had throughout the trial.

Pocock: It's not for me to say, but it was a fascinating trip to Glasgow every six months, with Michael chairing our data monitoring committee and I think the main issue, which Chris mentioned briefly, was that in the background there was some terrible newspaper coverage about low cholesterol causing cancer going on at the time, which at one point we thought would seriously damage the trial. I think the other thing about a data monitoring committee is that it is more important who you have on it than what your boundaries are for when you stop. I think Michael nurtured us through some exciting times, because we were seeing these dramatic benefits and I think that before the end, we had crossed any efficacy stopping boundary for benefit. But given the concerns about noncardiovascular deaths, we decided to go beyond such a boundary and I think that meant that as a result we got much more exciting solid evidence that had been pulled out earlier. The other thing is the benefit of having such trials independently run and it was Squibb who made that possible and, indeed, we should definitely encourage more companies in more fields nowadays to allow trials to be completely independent of their own company.

Durrington: I think those early statin trials were very courageous: 4S undoubtedly was, because at the time it was designed, many authoritative articles were saying that secondary prevention would be hopeless with cholesterol-lowering drugs.[266] It wasn't just the statin drugs themselves that were important in proving this wrong. I think it was also the fact that clinical trial design had reached a pinnacle of perfection. It had been informed by the mistakes of earlier trials, like the WHO clofibrate trial and people knew a lot of the pitfalls. The blood pressure trials had helped as well, so the statin trials coincided with greater knowledge of how to conduct a clinical trial, how to do the power calculations and all the rest of it, which I think was critical. Another important aspect was the intention-to-treat analysis, briefly mentioned by Chris [Packard].[267] One of the problems you [Michael Oliver] had with the WHO trial was that we never really got to grips with the actual results, because the intention-to-treat analysis was published only in a letter to the *Lancet* about ten years after the trial was finished.[268] Although we were led to believe that there was this increase in noncardiovascular mortality in the main report, I am not sure whether there really was. Despite subsequent fibrate trials, such as Veterans Affairs High Density Lipoprotein Cholesterol Intervention Trial (VAHIT), for historical reasons we unfortunately still need another convincing fibrate trial.[269] I think we may get it with the Fenofibrate Intervention and Event Lowering in Diabetes (FIELD) study: we need more evidence before we can know whether that fascinating group of drugs actually does any good, overall.[270]

Oliver: Well, Jerry Morris and I sweated blood about that letter, but we had to publish it, and nobody was going to accept another article, because the main results had already been published.

Morris: I think it was a nightmare. I would say that we knew little, at least I knew little, about such structure of a clinical trial in the middle 1960s.

Galton: Just a comment about the early origin of statins.[271] Another great missed British opportunity arose, because Beechams had the franchise for the early

---

[266] Scandinavian Simvastatin Survival Study (4S) (1994).

[267] Califf (2002).

[268] Heady *et al.* (1992).

[269] Rubins *et al.* for the Veterans Affairs High-Density Lipoprotein Cholesterol Intervention Trial Study Group (1999).

[270] Keech *et al.* for FIELD study investigators (2005).

[271] Endo *et al.* (1977).

fungal metabolite, which they called compactin.[272] John Reckless with a great deal of enterprise – I am only sorry he is not here today – managed to get some from Beechams and actually showed that it inhibited HMG-CoA reductase in leucocytes from normal and FH patients. Perhaps John [Betteridge] might like to talk about this, since he did some of the experiments.[273] But compactin gave a lot of complications *in vivo*, so Beechams sold it to Merck, Sharpe and Dohme, who developed lovastatin and the others from it.[274]

Davey Smith: I wanted to ask people who were around at the time about the clofibrate issue, as it has been mentioned frequently. If this meeting was in the US and people were talking about the slow introduction of cholesterol drugs, they would discuss triparanol (otherwise known as MER 29) that was introduced as an effective cholesterol-lowering agent and marketed very strongly in the US in the early 1960s.[275] However, it caused serious eye problems and there was some suggestion of increased death. Surely the triparanol story was something that inhibited the introduction of these drugs without trial evidence? It wasn't marketed in Britain, perhaps because triparanol was MER 29 and MER 30 was thalidomide.[276]

Packard: It was a huge issue when we were designing the WOSCOPS study. Everybody who was randomized and everybody who went to the end of year 1 had to undergo corneal screening. We used every ophthalmologist in the west of Scotland. After the first year we went back to the Food and Drug Administration (US FDA) and said, 'There's no issue here' and fortunately they accepted that. They released us from what would have been annual corneal screens.

Sanders: I want to make a comment really about lifestyle modification trials, which basically starred diet, smoking, blood pressure, and they really have been a total failure on an individual basis, compared with the drug trials. But if we look at changes that have occurred in the food chain which haven't involved individual choice, what has happened is that saturated fat intake has fallen by about 20 per cent down to about 12 per cent. The average blood cholesterol level in the population has fallen, even if you allow for changes in methodology, and

---

[272] Brown *et al.* (1976).

[273] Betteridge *et al.* (1978).

[274] The development of lovastatin is described in Appendix 2, pages 85–6.

[275] Fine (1972).

[276] For the background to the thalidomide tragedy, see Tansey and Reynolds (eds) (1997): 106–30.

CHD incidence has fallen. So I think although the drug trials demonstrate very clear effects, we can also see effects where changes in the food chain and changes in things like smoking prevalence have occurred.[277] They occur not because of the individual choice, they occur because of polity changes in society.

Thompson: I was just going to respond to the triparanol story by saying that the first homozygote that we ever plasma-exchanged had bilateral cataracts removed because she had been treated with triparanol.[278] And certainly in the days when we were using statin on a named-patient basis, we had to get the ophthalmologists to look at their lenses every month.

Oliver: Well I think we probably have covered quite a lot of the history. Anyone burning to say anything? I am sorry that one or two of the key people haven't been able to come, but many of you have provided additional information. I am very grateful to you and I hope that you have enjoyed it as much as I have.

Booth: On behalf of Tilli Tansey, I would like to thank you for coming to this exciting meeting. I have been an observer at these meetings for many years, and one can always tell how successful they are by the number of people who leave after tea. I don't think anybody did today and the discussion has been lively, encouraging and extremely interesting. I think we should thank Dr Daphne Christie for all the hard work she has done with Michael Oliver in organizing this meeting.

We have been discussing a British disease, first described, if you didn't know this, in 1776, when the surgeon John Hunter, whose patient had died suddenly with angina pectoris, reported of the heart that the coronary arteries from their origins upon their aorta and to their ratifications upon the heart surface were converted to one piece of bone.[279] To my knowledge, that is the first description of CHD.

I think finally we should thank Michael Oliver, who has been a wonderful Chairman; he has done a great deal of work.

---

[277] Principal Investigators (1978); Multiple Risk Factor Intervention Trial Research Group (1982). The intervention trials have been systematically reviewed by Hooper *et al.* (2001a and b). Responses, Mann *et al.* (2001) Hu *et al.* (2001), with reply by Hooper *et al.* (2001c).

[278] See Glossary, page 146.

[279] Elliot (1782). See also Morgagni (1762): xxiii, xxvi, xxvii.

Appendix 1

The 'diet–heart' hypothesis by Gerry Shaper

I was and am still concerned that the 'diet–heart' hypothesis, which is deeply entrenched and widely accepted in the statements of the American Heart Association and other North American bodies, has not been endorsed or denied by British authorities but allowed to float in the background without any firm statement being made by major official bodies, government or other.

The 'diet–heart' hypothesis states that a particular type of diet (specifically one high in saturated fatty acids) leads to high levels of blood cholesterol in individuals and populations and that this phenomenon is the necessary (essential) factor for increasing susceptibility to atherosclerosis and CHD in populations, although it may not be sufficient by itself to produce CHD. All other factors, such as tobacco smoking, physical inactivity and diabetes mellitus, are aggravating factors. However, if there is not a high blood cholesterol level, these factors, however injurious to other systems and conditions, have a small impact on the risk of CHD in a population. In this model, CHD is affected by a wide variety of genetic and environmental factors (i.e. it is multifactorial) but the dietary factors leading to a high blood cholesterol level are fundamental and necessary for a high level of CHD in a population. There are, of course, conditions in which a high blood cholesterol in individuals is not dietary in origin – for example in familial hypercholesterolaemia and chronic renal failure – but this does not negate the concept as applied to populations.

In the UK, the concept of CHD as a multifactorial disease is widely accepted and forms the basis of most scientific research and public health action towards the prevention of CHD. However, the term multifactorial is interpreted and used as meaning that atherosclerosis and CHD can arise from many different causes, usually in combination, rather than that there is any one fundamental (essential) cause for the condition in a population.

It is the history of this hypothesis, its promulgation and its dissemination, and the opposition, scientific and political, to the hypothesis that require to be discussed and documented.

Personal comment

My first period in the UK was in 1953–56 inclusive, first in Liverpool and then at the Hammersmith in London as Registrar to Sir John McMichael and

Professor John Shillingford. The research emphasis was on clinical cardiology and catheters, and there was little interest in the nature of atherosclerosis, in the lipid hypothesis or in possible nutritional aspects of cardiovascular disease. Coming from a medical school (Cape Town), where interethnic studies in blood lipids and cardiovascular disease (Bronte-Stewart), nutrition and chronic disease (Brock, see Figure 1) and coagulation and fibrinolysis (Merskey) were in full swing, with stimulating visits from Ancel Keys and other American workers, the lack of interest in this area in the UK was marked and disappointing. The atmosphere in the UK at that time was hostile to the American views on nutrition as a fundamental factor in atherosclerosis.

There followed a long period in Uganda with work in different ethnic groups (African, Asian, European) on lipid patterns, body build, coagulation and fibrinolysis and studies in nomadic groups of blood lipids and blood pressure.[280] At this time, in the early 1960s, work was also emerging from South Africa, Ceylon, Polynesia and New Guinea as well as East Africa about lipids, coagulation, platelet behaviour and fibrinolysis, with important UK contributions from Fearnley and Chakrabarti (fibrinolysis) and from Helen Payling Wright (platelet adhesiveness).[281]

It became apparent from the international studies that body weight, blood pressure and blood lipids did not necessarily increase with increasing age, and that levels regarded as 'normal' in Western societies were not 'biologically normal', that is, conducive to a healthy vasculature and an absence of atherosclerotic disease. In addition, in populations with low blood lipids, fibrinolytic activity was very marked compared with groups with higher blood lipids and with a high risk of cardiovascular disease.

I returned to the UK in 1970 to join Jerry Morris' MRC Social Medicine Unit, where there was a major focus on CHD with interests ranging from all aspects of physical activity, to the effects of water hardness, of diet, regional variations in cardiovascular disease (CVD) and drug treatments for lowering blood cholesterol levels. With Jean Marr, we studied the effects of dietary change on blood cholesterol levels in civil servants and showed that, without recourse to strict diets or to the family, these men were able to make significant and sustained reductions to their cholesterol levels over a four-year period.

---

[280] Shaper *et al.* (1963, 1966).

[281] Chakrabarti and Fearnley (1962); Wright (1941). See note 90.

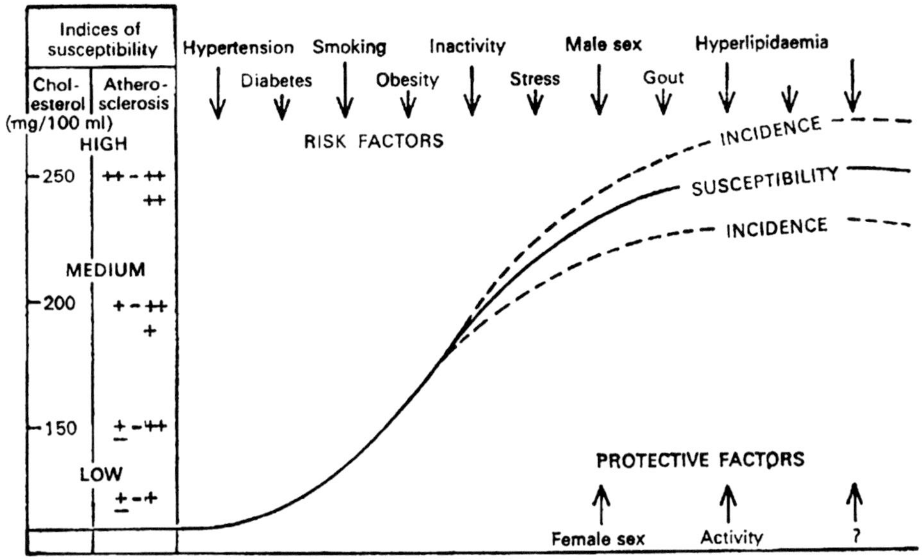

Figure 6: A model of community susceptibility and the incidence of CHD, 1972.
From Shaper (1972): 297.

The RCP/BCS Report

A key happening at this time was the setting up of a Joint Working Party of the Royal College of Physicians of London and the British Cardiac Society on prevention of coronary heart disease, brought about by Keith Ball and Dick Turner and including in its membership Michael Oliver, Geoffrey Rose, John Goodwin, Walter Somerville and others, and with contributions to the report from Harry Keen and Hugh Tunstall-Pedoe.[282] The report was published in 1976 and was distributed by the Chief Medical Officer [Sir Henry Yellowlees] to all doctors in the UK. There is little in the report that would not be acceptable today, with a focus on diet and with dietary recommendations for the whole community.

At this time, there were prominent individuals in British cardiology who vigorously opposed the dissemination of this report, and throughout the late 1970s, 1980s and into the 1990s, there was continued concern that lowering blood cholesterol by any means, including dietary change, might have a deleterious effect on human biological systems. The implication has been that

[282] Royal College of Physicians of London and the British Cardiac Society (1976).

lower blood cholesterol levels, however achieved, might be dangerous. It is of considerable interest to note that these concerns have not subsided, and with the widespread use of drugs for lowering blood lipids, there is renewed concern in this direction.

Observational population studies

In 1975, the MRC awarded a programme grant for studying the regional variations in cardiovascular disease with a particular interest in the effects of water quality (softness and hardness) and this study developed into the British Regional Heart Study (BRHS) involving some 8 000 middle-aged men in 24 British towns.[283] It rapidly emerged that blood lipid levels were uniformly high in every town studied, so that risk related to blood lipids was equally high everywhere in Britain. Variations in prevalence and incidence were related to the other risk factors, which varied considerably from town to town. The BRHS has continued to the present day and has made contributions to many aspects of cardiovascular disease, including observations on diabetes, the Metabolic Syndrome, overweight and obesity and physical activity, and with studies extending to children and women throughout the UK.

[283] For details and full bibliography of the British Regional Heart Study, recruited in 1978–80, see www.ucl.ac.uk/primcare-popsci/brhs (visited 12 January 2006).

Appendix 2

The discovery and development of lovastatin by Jonathan Tobert[284]

Inhibitors of HMG-CoA reductase (statins) are widely prescribed, and one, simvastatin, can now be obtained without a prescription in the UK. However, the development of the first member of the class, lovastatin, was far from straightforward.

HMG-CoA reductase is the rate-limiting enzyme in the cholesterol biosynthetic pathway. Natural products with a powerful inhibitory effect on HMG-CoA reductase, including ML236B (compactin), were first discovered by the Japanese microbiologist Akira Endo.[285] The compound was highly effective in reducing LDL cholesterol in patients with heterozygous familial hypercholesterolaemia (FH).[286] In 1978, Alberts, Chen and others at Merck Research Laboratories found a potent inhibitor of HMG-CoA reductase in a fermentation broth of *Aspergillus terreus*, which they named mevinolin; later, the official name (US Adopted Name or USAN) was established as lovastatin.[287]

Merck began clinical trials of lovastatin in healthy volunteers in April 1980. Lovastatin was shown to be remarkably effective for lowering LDL cholesterol in healthy volunteers, with no obvious adverse effects.[288] However, this encouraging start was soon interrupted. For reasons that have never been made public (but which were believed to include serious animal toxicity), clinical trials with compactin were stopped by its developer Sankyo in September 1980. Because of the close structural similarity between compactin and lovastatin, Merck promptly suspended clinical studies with lovastatin, and initiated additional

---

[284] Prepared by Dr Jonathan Tobert at the request of Professor Oliver for the Witness Seminar held on 8 March 2005, based on Tobert (2003).

[285] Endo *et al.* (1976b, 1977).

[286] Mabuchi *et al.* (1981).

[287] Alberts *et al.* (1980). The USAN of a drug can be found in the *US Pharmacopeia (USP) Dictionary of US Adopted Names and International Drug Names*, which contains US adopted names, official drug names for the USP and the National Formulary, previously used official names, international and nonproprietary names, British approved names, Japanese approved names, miscellaneous older names, and trade names. See www.cas.org/ONLINE/DBSS/usanss.html (visited 25 January 2006).

[288] Tobert *et al.* (1982a and b).

animal safety studies. The viability of the drug was in serious doubt. However, in 1982 studies resumed outside Merck in a small number of patients with severe FH refractory to existing therapy; they showed dramatic reductions in LDL cholesterol with very few adverse effects.[289]

In 1983, after the additional animal safety studies with lovastatin revealed no toxicity of the type believed to be associated with compactin, Merck decided to re-initiate the clinical development programme, initially in patients at very high risk of MI. Because of concerns about patient safety, this was a difficult decision. Notwithstanding the excellent tolerability to date in small, short-term clinical studies, it was quite possible that more clinical experience, as well as long-term animal toxicology studies, would uncover serious safety issues.

In randomized, double-blind phase IIb placebo-controlled studies, lovastatin was as effective in patients with heterozygous FH and patients with CHD and nonfamilial hypercholesterolaemia as it had been in healthy volunteers.[290] In larger phase III studies, lovastatin produced much greater reductions in LDL cholesterol than the control agents cholestyramine and probucol, with very few adverse effects.[291] There was a profound reduction of apolipoprotein B-containing lipoproteins, especially LDL cholesterol (average reduction of 40 per cent at the maximal dose of 80mg daily) and, to a lesser extent, plasma triglycerides, together with a small increase in HDL cholesterol. Observed tolerability continued to be excellent, with very few patients withdrawing from treatment due to adverse effects. In November 1986, Merck applied for regulatory approval of lovastatin, which was obtained on 31 August 1987 from the US FDA; Merck had patent rights only in certain other countries, all of which later granted approval. More details on the complex history of lovastatin (and other statins), including the evaluation of potential and actual adverse effects, may be found in a recent review.[292]

---

[289] Bilheimer *et al.* (1983); Illingworth and Sexton (1984).

[290] Havel *et al.* (1987); Lovastatin Study Group II (1986); Tobert *et al.* (1982b).

[291] Lovastatin Study Group III (1988); Lovastatin Study Group IV (1990).

[292] Tobert (2003).

References

Adams C W, Bayliss O B, Ibrahim M Z. (1963) The distribution of lipids and enzymes in the aortic wall in dietary rabbit atheroma and human atherosclerosis. *Journal of Pathology and Bacteriology* **86:** 421–30.

Alberts A W, Chen J, Kuron G, Hunt V, Huff J, Hoffman C, Rothrock J, Lopez M, Joshua H, Harris E, Patchett A, Monaghan R, Currie S, Stapley E, Albers-Schonberg G, Hensens O, Hirshfield J, Hoogsteen K, Liesch J, Springer J. (1980) Mevinolin: a highly potent competitive inhibitor of hydroxymethylglutaryl-coenzyme A reductase and a cholesterol-lowering agent. *Proceedings of the National Academy of Sciences of the USA* **77:** 3957–61.

Albrink M J. (1964) Clinical evaluation of drugs for the treatment of diabetes. *Diabetes* **13:** 429–30.

Albrink M J, Man E B. (1958) Serum triglycerides in health and diabetes. *Diabetes* **7:** 194–201.

Albrink M J, Lavietes P H, Man E B. (1963) Vascular disease and serum lipids in diabetes mellitus. Observations over 30 years (1931–61). *Annals of Internal Medicine* **58:** 305–23.

Anderson J T, Aresu M, Biorck G, Brock J F, Bronte-Stewart B, Del Vecchio A, Fidanza F, Keys A, Keys M H, Malmros H, Poppi A, Posteli T, Swahn B. (1956) Physical activity and the diet in populations differing in serum cholesterol. *Journal of Clinical Investigation* **35:** 1173–81.

Anitschkov N, Chalatow S. (1913) [On experimental cholesterin steatosis and its significance in the origin of some pathological processes.] German. *Zentralblatt fur Allgemeine Pathologie und Pathologische Anatomie* **24:** 1–9. Reproduced as Anon. (1983).

Anonymous. (1968) Hubert Maitland Turnbull. *Munk's Roll* **5:** 425–6.

Anonymous. (1975a) Letter: does polyunsaturated fat beef work? *Medical Journal of Australia* **2:** 68–9.

Anonymous. (1975b) Editorial: polyunsaturated beef-eaters. *Lancet* **ii:** 960–1.

Anonymous. (1983) Classics in arteriosclerosis research: On experimental cholesterin steatosis and its significance in the origin of some pathological processes by N Anitschkov and S Chalatow, translated by Mary Z Pelias, 1913. *Arteriosclerosis* **3:** 178–82.

Anonymous. (1996) Frontiers of atherosclerosis and lipoprotein research. Special issue in memory of Professor Shlomo Eisenberg. *Israel Journal of Medical Sciences* **32:** i, 345–508.

Aro A, Tuomilehto J, Kostiainen E, Uusitalo U, Pietinen P. (1987) Boiled coffee increases serum low density lipoprotein concentration. *Metabolism* **36:** 1027–30.

Astrup T. (1956) Fibrinolysis in the organism. *Blood* **11:** 781–806.

Austin M A, King M C, Vranizan K M, Krauss R M. (1990) Atherogenic lipoprotein phenotype. A proposed genetic marker for coronary heart disease risk. *Circulation* **82:** 495–506.

Austin M A, Breslow J L, Hennekens C H, Buring J E, Willett W C, Krauss R M. (1988) Low-density lipoprotein subclass patterns and risk of myocardial infarction. *Journal of the American Medical Association* **260:** 1917–21.

Barker D J P. (1972) *Practical Epidemiology*. Edinburgh: Churchill Livingstone.

Barker D J P, Osmond C. (1986) Infant mortality, childhood nutrition, and ischaemic heart disease in England and Wales. *Lancet* **i:** 1077–81.

Barker D J P, Rose G. (1976, 1979, 1984, 1990) *Epidemiology in Medical Practice*. Edinburgh; New York, NY: Churchill Livingstone.

Barker D J P, Eriksson J G, Forsen T, Osmond C. (2002) Fetal origins of adult disease: strength of effects and biological basis. *International Journal of Epidemiology* **31:** 1235–9.

Barker D J P, Winter P D, Osmond C, Margetts B, Simmonds S J. (1989) Weight in infancy and death from ischaemic heart disease. *Lancet* **ii:** 577–80.

Barr D P, Russ E M. (1951) Protein-lipid relationships in diabetes mellitus. *Transactions of the Association of American Physicians* **64:** 297–303.

Barr D P, Russ E M, Eder H A. (1951) Protein-lipid relationships in human plasma. II. In atherosclerosis and related conditions. *American Journal of Medicine* **11:** 480–93.

Berridge V, Christie D A, Tansey E M (eds) (2006) Public health in the 1980s and 1990s: Decline and rise? *Wellcome Witnesses to Twentieth Century Medicine,* volume 26, London: The Wellcome Trust Centre for the History of Medicine at UCL. Freely available online at www.ucl.ac.uk/histmed following the links to Publications/Wellcome Witnesses.

Betteridge D J, Krone W, Reckless J P, Galton D J. (1978) Compactin inhibits cholesterol synthesis in lymphocytes and intestinal mucosa from patients with familial hypercholesterolaemia. *Lancet* **ii:** 1342–3.

Bilheimer D W, Grundy S M, Brown M S, Goldstein J L. (1983) Mevinolin and colestipol stimulate receptor-mediated clearance of low density lipoprotein from plasma in familial hypercholesterolemia heterozygotes. *Proceedings of the National Academy of Sciences of the USA* **80:** 4124–8.

Blackhart B D, Ludwig E M, Pierotti V R, Caiati L, Onasch M A, Wallis S C, Powell L, Pease R, Knott T J, Chu M-L, Mahley R W, Scott J, McCarthy B J, Levy-Wilson B. (1986) Structure of the human apolipoprotein B gene. *Journal of Biological Chemistry* **261:** 15364–7.

Blankenhorn D H, Nessim S A, Johnson R L, Sanmarco M E, Azen S P, Cashin-Hemphill L. (1987) Beneficial effects of combined colestipol-niacin therapy on coronary atherosclerosis and coronary venous bypass grafts. *Journal of the American Medical Association* **257:** 3233–40. Erratum in: *JAMA* (1988) **259:** 2698.

Born G V R. (2002) Afterword: Platelets, a personal story, in Gresele P, Page C P, Fuster V, Vermylen J. (eds) *Platelets in Thrombotic and Non-thrombotic Disorders: Pathophysiology, Pharmacology and Therapeutics.* Cambridge and New York: Cambridge University Press, 1063–72.

Born G V R. (2003) Update on platelets: a personal story. *Platelets* **14:** 333–4.

Born G V R, Palinski W. (1985) Unusually high concentrations of sialic acids on the surface of vascular endothelia. *British Journal of Experimental Pathology* **66:** 543–49.

Born G V R, Medina R, Shafi S, Cardona-Sanclemente L E. (2003) Factors influencing the uptake of atherogenic plasma proteins by artery walls. *Biorheology* **40:** 13–22.

Böttcher C J. (1967) Chemical factors in atherogenesis. *Pathologia et Microbiologia* (Basel) **30:** 619–28.

Boyd G S. (1954) The estimation of serum lipoproteins; a micromethod based on zone electrophoresis and cholesterol estimations. *Biochemical Journal* **58:** 680–5.

Boyd G S, Oliver M F. (1956) Endocrine aspects of coronary sclerosis. *Lancet* **ii:** 1273–6.

Brenner S. (2001). *My Life in Science*. London: BioMed Central.

Brensike J F, Levy R I, Kelsey S F, Passamani E R, Richardson J M, Loh I K, Stone N J, Aldrich R F, Battaglini J W, Moriarty D J, Fisher M R, Friedman L, Friedewald W, Detre K M, Epstein S E. (1984) Effects of therapy with cholestyramine on progression of coronary arteriosclerosis: results of the NHLBI Type II Coronary Intervention Study. *Circulation* **69:** 313–24.

Bronte-Stewart B. (1965) Certain etiologic aspects of atherosclerosis. *Angiology* **16:** 427–32.

Bronte-Stewart B, Keys A, Brock J F. (1955) Serum-cholesterol, diet, and coronary heart disease; an inter-racial survey in the Cape Peninsula. *Lancet* **269:** 1103–8.

Bronte-Stewart B, Antonis A, Eales L, Brock J F. (1956) Effects of feeding different fats on serum-cholesterol level. *Lancet* **270:** 521–6.

Brown A G, Smale T C, King T J, Hasenkamp R, Thompson R H. (1976) Crystal and molecular structure of compactin, a new antifungal metabolite from *Penicillium brevicompactum*. *Journal of the Chemical Society* [Perkin 1]: 1165–70.

Brown G, Albers J J, Fisher L D, Schaefer S M, Lin J T, Kaplan C, Zhao X Q, Bisson B D, Fitzpatrick V F, Dodge H T. (1990) Regression of coronary artery disease as a result of intensive lipid-lowering therapy in men with high levels of apolipoprotein B. *New England Journal of Medicine* **323:** 1289–98.

Brunt J N, Watts G F, Lewis B, Smith L D, Coltart D J. (1995) Quantitative coronary cineangiography for the study of atherosclerosis. *Medical Engineering and Physics* **17:** 356–65.

Buchwald H, Varco R L, Matts J P, Long J M, Fitch L L, Campbell G S, Pearce M B, Yellin A E, Edmiston W A, Smink R D Jr, *et al.* (1990) Effect of partial ileal bypass surgery on mortality and morbidity from coronary heart disease in patients with hypercholesterolemia. Report of the Program on the Surgical Control of the Hyperlipidemias (POSCH). *New England Journal of Medicine* **323:** 946–55.

Burr M L, Fehily A M, Gilbert J F, Rogers S, Holliday R M, Sweetnam P M, Elwood P C, Deadman N M. (1989) Effects of changes in fat, fish and fibre intakes on death and myocardial reinfarction: diet and reinfarction trial (DART). *Lancet* **ii:** 757–61.

Califf R M. (2002) Chapter 15. Large clinical trials in clinical research institutes. In Gallin J I. (ed.) *Principles and Practice of Clinical Research*. San Diego, CA: Academic Press, 225–50.

Carstairs K C, Woolf N, Crawford T. (1964) Immunohistochemical cross-reaction between platelets and fibrin. *Journal of Pathology and Bacteriology* **88:** 537–40.

Carter C O, Slack J, Myant N B. (1971) Genetics of hyperlipoproteinaemias. *Lancet* **i:** 400–1.

Chakrabarti R, Fearnley G R. (1962) The 'fibrinolytic potential' as a simple measure of spontaneous fibrinolysis. *Journal of Clinical Pathology* **15:** 228–30.

Chakrabarti R, Bielawiec M, Evans J F, Fearnley G R. (1968) Methodological study and a recommended technique for determining the euglobulin lysis time. *Journal of Clinical Pathology* **21:** 698–701.

Chave S P, Morris J N, Moss S, Semmence A M. (1978) Vigorous exercise in leisure time and the death rate: a study of male civil servants. *Journal of Epidemiology and Community Health* **32:** 239–43.

Christensen B, Glueck C, Kwiterovich P, Degroot I, Chase G, Heiss G, Mowery R, Tamir I, Rifkind B. (1980) Plasma cholesterol and triglyceride distributions in 13 665 children and adolescents: the Prevalence Study of the Lipid Research Clinics Program. *Pediatric Research* **14:** 194–202.

Christie D A, Tansey E M. (eds) (2003) Genetic Testing. *Wellcome Witnesses to Twentieth Century Medicine*, vol. 17. London: Wellcome Trust Centre for the History of Medicine at UCL. Freely available from www.ucl.ac.uk/histmed/ following links to Publications/Wellcome Witnesses.

Clifton-Bligh P, Galton D J. (1976) The esterification of exogenous fatty acids by adipose tissue of hypertriglyceridaemic subjects with or without diabetes mellitus. *Clinical Science and Molecular Medicine* **51:** 257–65.

Cohen J, Pertsemlidis A, Kotowski I K, Graham R, Garcia C K, Hobbs H H. (2005) Low LDL cholesterol in individuals of African descent resulting from frequent nonsense mutations in PCSK9. *Nature Genetics* **37:** 161–5. Epub Jan 16 2005. Erratum in: *Nature Genetics* **37:** 328.

Cook R P. (ed.) (1958) *Cholesterol: Chemistry, biochemistry and pathology*. New York, NY: Academic Press.

Corbishley C, Burke M. (2003) Obituary: Michael John Davies. *British Medical Journal* **326:** 1270.

Cornforth J W. (1959) Biosynthesis of fatty acids and cholesterol considered as chemical processes. *Journal of Lipid Research* **1:** 3–28.

Cornforth J W. (1973) The logic of working with enzymes. *Chemical Society Reviews* **2:** 1–20.

Cornforth J W, Youthotsky I, Popják G. (1954) Absolute configuration of cholesterol. *Nature* **173:** 536.

Cottet J, Mathivat A, Redel J. (1954) Therapeutic study of a synthetic hypocholesterolaemic agent: phenyl ethyl acetic acid. *La Presse Medicale* **62:** 939–41.

Crepaldi G. (1971) [Relations between diet and atherosclerosis] Italian. *Minerva Medica* **62:** 3433–51.

Dangerfield W G, Smith E B. (1955) An investigation of serum lipids and lipoproteins by paper electrophoresis. *Journal of Clinical Pathology* **8:** 132–9.

Davey Smith G. (2004) A conversation with Jerry Morris. *Epidemiology* **15:** 770–3.

Davey Smith G, Ebrahim S. (2003) 'Mendelian randomization': can genetic epidemiology contribute to understanding environmental determinants of disease? *International Journal of Epidemiology* **32:** 1–22.

Davey Smith G, Nutbeam D. (1988) Public attitudes and knowledge regarding coronary heart disease. In Catford J C. (ed.) *Coronary Heart Disease Prevention: Action in the UK 1984–87*. London: National Forum for CHD Prevention, 97–102.

Davey Smith G, Pekkanen J. (1992a) Should there be a moratorium on the use of cholesterol-lowering drugs? *British Medical Journal* **304:** 431–4.

Davey Smith G, Pekkanen J. (1992b) The cholesterol controversy. *British Medical Journal* **304:** 913.

Davey Smith G, Shipley M J. (1989) Plasma cholesterol concentration and primary brain tumours. *British Medical Journal* **299:** 26–7.

Davey Smith G, Song F, Sheldon T A. (1993) Cholesterol lowering and mortality: the importance of considering initial level of risk. *British Medical Journal* **306:** 1367–73.

Davey Smith G, Shipley M J, Marmot M G, Rose G. (1992a) Plasma cholesterol concentration and mortality. The Whitehall Study. *Journal of the American Medical Association* **267:** 70–6.

Davey Smith G, Neaton J D, Ben-Shlomo Y, Shipley M, Wentworth D. (1992b) Serum cholesterol concentration and primary malignant brain tumors: a prospective study. *American Journal of Epidemiology* **135:** 259–65.

Davey Smith G, Hart C, Blane D, Gillis C, Hawthorne V. (1997) Lifetime socioeconomic position and mortality: prospective observational study. *British Medical Journal* **314:** 547–52. Erratum in *BMJ* (1997) **314:** 1012.

Davies M J. (1992) Anatomic features in victims of sudden coronary death. Coronary artery pathology. *Circulation* **85:** I19–24.

Davies M J. (1996) Stability and instability: two faces of coronary atherosclerosis. The Paul Dudley White Lecture 1995. *Circulation* **94:** 2013–20.

Davies M J, Thomas A C. (1985) Plaque fissuring – the cause of acute myocardial infarction, sudden ischaemic death, and crescendo angina. *British Heart Journal* **53:** 363–73.

Davies, M J, Woolf N, Robertson W B. (1976) Pathology of acute myocardial infarction with particular reference to occlusive coronary thrombi. *British Heart Journal* **38:** 659–64.

Davies M J, Woolf N, Rowles P, Richardson P D. (1994) Lipid and cellular constituents of unstable human aortic plaques. *Basic Research in Cardiology* **89:** 33–9.

de Gennes J L, Touraine R, Maunand B, Truffert J, Laudat P. (1967) [Homozygous cutaneo-tendinous forms of hypercholesteremic xanthomatosis in an exemplary familial case. Trial of plasmapheresis an heroic treatment.] French. *Bulletins et memoires de la Sociéte médicale des hopitaux de Paris* **118:** 1377–402.

Department of Health and Social Security (DHSS), Committee on Medical Aspects of Food Policy, Panel on Diet in Relation to Cardiovascular Disease (COMA). (1984) *Diet and Cardiovascular Disease: Report of the Panel on Diet in Relation to Cardiovascular Disease.* Health and social subjects series No. 28. London: HMSO.

Dollery C. (1995) Sir John McMichael 1904–93. *Biographical Memoirs of Fellows of the Royal Society* **41:** 283–96.

Drury A N, Grant R T. (1945–48) Sir Thomas Lewis. *Obituary Notices of Fellows of the Royal Society* **5:** 179–202.

Duffield R G, Lewis B, Miller N E, Jamieson C W, Brunt J N, Colchester A C. (1983) Treatment of hyperlipidaemia retards progression of symptomatic femoral atherosclerosis. A randomized controlled trial. *Lancet* **ii:** 639–42.

Durrington P N. (2003) Chapter 16. Gender and coronary heart disease. In Durrington P N, Mackness M I, Miller J P, Rees A. (eds). *Year in Dyslipidaemia 2003.* Oxford: Clinical Publishing, 297–306.

Durrington P N. (2004) Statin policy and target populations: evidence-based or evidence-biased? *Current Opinion in Lipidology* **15:** 381–6.

Edington J D, Geekie M, Carter R, Benfield L, Ball M, Mann J. (1989) Serum lipid response to dietary cholesterol in subjects fed a low-fat, high-fiber diet. *American Journal of Clinical Nutrition* **50:** 58–62.

Eisenberg S, Bilheimer D W, Levy R I, Lindgren F T. (1973) On the metabolic conversion of human plasma very low density lipoprotein to low density lipoprotein. *Biochimica et Biophysica Acta* **326:** 361–77.

Elliot J. (1782) *A Complete Collection of the Medical and Philosophical Works of John Fothergill with an Account of his Life; and Occasional Notes.* London: G Robinson: 531–6.

Endo A, Kuroda M, Tsujita Y. (1976a) ML-236A, ML-236B, and ML-236C, new inhibitors of cholesterogenesis produced by *Penicillium citrinium. Journal of Antibiotics* **29:** 1346–8.

Endo A, Kuroda M, Tanzawa K. (1976b) Competitive inhibition of 3-hydroxy-3-methylglutaryl coenzyme A reductase by ML-236A and ML-236B fungal metabolites, having hypocholesterolaemic activity. *FEBS Letters* **72:** 323–4.

Endo A, Tsujita Y, Kuroda M, Tanzawa K. (1977) Inhibition of cholesterol synthesis *in vitro* and *in vivo* by ML-236A and ML-236B, competitive inhibitors of 3-hydroxy-3-methylglutaryl-coenzyme A reductase. *European Journal of Biochemistry* **77:** 31–6.

Evans W. (1948) *Diseases of the Heart and Arteries.* Edinburgh; London: E and S Livingstone.

Ewin J H. (2001) *Fine Wines and Fish Oils: The Life of Hugh Macdonald Sinclair.* Oxford: Oxford University Press.

Fehily A M, Pickering J E, Yarnell J W, Elwood P C. (1994) Dietary indices of atherogenicity and thrombogenicity and ischaemic heart disease risk: the Caerphilly Prospective Study. *British Journal of Nutrition* **71:** 249–57.

Fernandez-Armesto F. (2001) *Food: A history.* London: Macmillan.

Fine R A. (1972) *The Great Drug Deception: The shocking story of MER 29 and the folks who gave you thalidomide.* New York, NY: Stein and Day.

Florey H. (ed.) (1970) *General Pathology.* 4th edn. London: Lloyd-Luke Medical Books Ltd.

Fogelman A M, Shechter I, Seager J, Hokom M, Child JS, Edwards P A. (1980) Malondialdehyde alteration of low density lipoproteins leads to cholesteryl ester accumulation in human monocyte-macrophages. *Proceedings of the National Academy of Sciences of the USA* **77:** 2214–18.

Foyle W J, Carstensen E, Fernandez M C, Yudkin J S. (1995) Longitudinal study of associations of microalbuminuria with the insulin resistance syndrome and sodium-lithium countertransport in nondiabetic subjects. *Arteriosclerosis, Thrombosis, and Vascular Biology* **15:** 1330–7.

Frantz I D Jr, Moore R B, (1969) The sterol hypothesis in atherogenesis. *American Journal of Medicine* **46:** 684–90.

Fredrickson D S, Lees R S. (1966) *The Metabolic Basis of Inherited Disease.* 2nd edn. New York, NY: McGraw-Hill. Chapter 22 on familial hyperlipoproteinaemia, pages 429–88.

Fredrickson D S, Levy R I, Lees R S. (1967) Fat transport in lipoproteins – an integrated approach to mechanisms and disorders. *New England Journal of Medicine* **276:** 34–42; 94–103 148–56; 215–25; 273–81.

French J E. (1958) Chapter 17: Atherosclerosis, in Florey H. (ed.) *General Pathology: Based on lectures delivered at the Sir William Dunn School of Pathology, University of Oxford.* 2nd edn. London: Lloyd-Luke (Medical Books) Ltd: 351–77.

Frick M H, Elo O, Haapa K, Heinonen O P, Heinsalmi P, Helo P, Huttunen J K, Kaitaniemi P, Koskinen P, Manninen V, Mäenpää H, Mälkönen M, Mänttäri M, Norola S, Pasternack A, Pikkarainen J, Romo M, Sjöblom T, Nikkilä E A. (1987) Helsinki Heart Study: primary-prevention trial with gemfibrozil in middle-aged men with dyslipidemia. Safety of treatment, changes in risk factors, and incidence of coronary heart disease. *New England Journal of Medicine* **317:** 1237–45.

Friedewald W T, Levy R I, Fredrickson D S. (1972) Estimation of the concentration of low-density lipoprotein cholesterol in plasma, without use of the preparative ultracentrifuge. *Clinical Chemistry* **18:** 499–502.

Fullerton H W, Davie W J, Anastasopoulos G. (1953) Relationship of alimentary lipaemia to blood coagulability. *British Medical Journal* **ii:** 250–3.

Fulton W F M. (1965) *The Coronary Arteries.* Springfield, IL: Charles C Thomas.

Fulton W F M. (1993) Pathological concepts in acute coronary thrombosis: relevance to treatment. *British Heart Journal* **70:** 403–8.

Furst A L, Greaves D A, Hawthorne V M, McCartney H, Stewart G T. (1972) Candidates for coronaries. *British Medical Journal* **iv**: 366–7.

Gaffney P J, Edgell T A, Whitton C M. (1999) The haemostatic balance – Astrup revisited. *Haemostasis* **29:** 58–71.

Galton D J. (2003) *Dyslipidaemia*. Edinburgh: Churchill Livingstone. [Revised and expanded edn of Galton D J, Krone W. (1990) *Hyperlipidaemia in Practice*. London: Gower Medical Publishing.]

Gertler M M, White P D. (1954) *Coronary Heart Disease in Young Adults: A multidisciplinary study*. With the aid, advice, and editorial assistance of E F Bland. Cambridge, MA: Harvard University Press for the Commonwealth Fund.

Gilbert M. (1991) *Churchill: A life*. London: William Heinemann.

Gofman J W, Lindgren F T, Elliot H. (1949) Ultracentrifugal studies of lipoproteins of human serum. *Journal of Biological Chemistry* **179:** 973–9.

Gofman J W, Jones H B, Lindgren F T, Lyon T P, Elliott H A, Strisower B. (1950) Blood lipids and human atherosclerosis. *Circulation* **5:** 161–78.

Gofman J W, Jones H B, Lyon IP, Lindgren F T, Strisower B, Colman D, Herring V. (1952) Blood lipids and human atherosclerosis. *Circulation* **5:** 119–34.

Goldstein J L, Brown M S. (1977) The low-density lipoprotein pathway and its relation with atherosclerosis. *Annual Review of Biochemistry* **46:** 897–930.

Goldstein J L, Hazzard W R, Schrott H G, Bierman E L, Motulsky A G. (1973a) Hyperlipidemia in coronary heart disease: 1. Lipid levels in 500 survivors of myocardial infarction. *Journal of Clinical Investigation* **52:** 1533–43.

Goldstein J L, Schrott H G, Hazzard W R, Bierman E L, Motulsky A G. (1973b) Hyperlipidemia in coronary heart disease: 2. Genetic analysis of lipid levels in 176 families and delineation of a new inherited disorder, combined hyperlipidemia. *Journal of Clinical Investigation* **52:** 1544–68.

Gordon T, Castelli W P, Hjortland M C, Kannel W B, Dawber T R. (1977) Predicting coronary heart disease in middle-aged older persons. The Framingham study. *Journal of the American Medical Association* **238:** 497–9.

Gordon T, Kannel W B, Castelli W P, Dawber T R. (1981) Lipoproteins, cardiovascular disease, and death. The Framingham study. *Archives of Internal Medicine* **141:** 1128–31.

Gould R G, Popják G. (1957) Biosynthesis of cholesterol *in vivo* and *in vitro* from DL-β-hydroxy-β-methyl-δ -[2-^{14}C]-valerolactone. *Biochemical Journal* **66:** 51P.

Grady D, Herrington D, Bittner V, Blumenthal R, Davidson M, Hlatky M, Hsia J, Hulley S, Herd A, Khan S, Kristin Newby L, Waters D, Vittinghoff E, Wenger N, for the HERS Research Group. (2002) Cardiovascular disease outcomes during 6.8 years of hormone therapy: Heart and Estrogen/Progestin Replacement Study Follow-up (HERS II). *Journal of the American Medical Association* **288:** 49–57.

Gray J, Booth C. (1994) Sir Harold Himsworth. *Munk's Roll* **9:** 238–41.

Grundy S M. (1991) George Lyman Duff Memorial Lecture. Multifactorial etiology of hypercholesterolemia. Implications for prevention of coronary heart disease. *Arteriosclerosis and Thrombosis* **11:** 1619–35.

H(ampton) J R. (1991) Obituary: J R A Mitchell. *British Medical Journal* **302:** 843.

Hart C L, Davey Smith G, Hole D J, Hawthorne V M. (1999) Alcohol consumption and mortality from all causes, coronary heart disease, and stroke: results from a prospective cohort study of Scottish men with 21 years of follow-up. *British Medical Journal* **318:** 1725–9.

Haust M D, More R H, Bencosme S A, Balis J U. (1967) Electron microscopic studies in human atherosclerosis extracellular elements in aortic dots and streaks. *Experimental and Molecular Pathology* **6:** 300–13.

Havel R J, Hunninghake D B, Illingworth D R, Lees R S, Stein E A, Tobert J A, Bacon S R, Bolognese J A, Frost P H, Lamkin G E, Lees A M, Leon A S, Gardner K, Johnson G, Mellies M J, Rhymer P A, Tun P. (1987) Lovastatin (mevinolin) in the treatment of heterozygous familial hypercholesterolemia. A multicenter study. *Annals of Internal Medicine* **107:** 609–15.

Hawthorne F. (2003) *The Merck Druggernaut: The inside story of a pharmaceutical giant.* Hoboken, NJ: John Wiley & Sons, Inc.

Hawthorne V M. (1977) Diet and coronary heart disease. *British Medical Journal* **ii:** 186–7.

Hawthorne V M, Gillis C R, Lorimer A R, Calvert F R, Walker T J. (1969) Blood pressure in a Scottish island community. *British Medical Journal* **iv:** 651–4.

Hazzard W R, Goldstein J L, Schrott M G, Motulsky A G, Bierman E L. (1973) Hyperlipidemia in coronary heart disease: 3. Evaluation of lipoprotein phenotypes of 156 genetically defined survivors of myocardial infarction. *Journal of Clinical Investigation* **52:** 1569–77.

Heady J A, Morris J N, Oliver M F. (1992) WHO clofibrate/cholesterol trial: clarifications. *Lancet* **340:** 1405–6.

Heart Protection Study Collaborative Group. (2002) MRC/BHF Heart Protection Study of cholesterol lowering with simvastatin in 20 536 high risk individuals: a randomized placebo-controlled trial. *Lancet* **360:** 7–22.

Hegsted M. (1959) Comparative studies on the effect of dietary fats on serum cholesterol levels. *Federation Proceedings* **18:** 52–4.

Heiberg A, Berg K. (1976) The inheritance of hyperlipoproteinaemia with xanthomatosis. A study of 132 kindreds. *Clinical Genetics* **9:** 203–33.

Hendriks H F, Weststrate J A, van Vliet T, Meijer G W. (1999) Spreads enriched with three different levels of vegetable oil sterols and the degree of cholesterol lowering in normocholesterolaemic and mildly hypercholesterolaemic subjects. *European Journal of Clinical Nutrition* **53:** 319–27.

Henriksen T, Mahoney E M, Steinberg D. (1981) Enhanced macrophage degradation of low density lipoprotein previously incubated with cultured endothelial cells: recognition by receptors for acetylated low density lipoproteins *Proceedings of the National Academy of Sciences of the USA* **78:** 6499–503.

Higgins I T, Cochrane A L, Thomas A J. (1963) Epidemiological studies of coronary disease. *British Journal of Preventive and Social Medicine* **17:** 153–65.

Himsworth H P. (1936) Diabetes mellitus: its differentiation into insulin-sensitive and insulin-insensitive types. *Lancet* **i:** 127–30.

Himsworth H P. (1982) Thomas Lewis and the development of support for clinical research. *The Pharos of Alpha Omega Alpha* **45:** 15–19.

Hoff H F, Heideman C L, Gotto A M Jr, Gaubatz J W. (1977) Apolipoprotein B retention in the grossly normal and atherosclerotic human aorta. *Circulation Research* **41:** 684–90.

Hofmann A F, Zöllner N. (2000) *Siegfried Thannhauser (1885–1962): Physician and scientist in turbulent times*. Freiburg: Falk Foundation.

Hooper L, Summerbell C D, Higgins J P T, Thompson R L, Clements G, Capps N, Davey Smith G, Riemersma R A, Ebrahim S. (2001a) Reduced or modified dietary fat for preventing cardiovascular disease. *Cochrane Database Systematic Review 2001* **(3):** CD002137.

Hooper L, Summerbell C D, Higgins J P, Thompson R L, Capps N E, Davey Smith G, Riemersma R A, Ebrahim S. (2001b) Dietary fat intake and prevention of cardiovascular disease: systematic review. *British Medical Journal* **322:** 757–63.

Hooper L, Summerbell C D, Thompson R L, Capps N E, Davey Smith G, Riemersma R A, Ebrahim S. (2001c) Author's reply. *British Medical Journal* **323:** 1001–2.

Howard A N, Patelski J, Bowyer D E, Gresham G A. (1972) Aortic lipolytic enzymes in atherosclerosis. *Biochemical Journal* **128:** 41P.

Hu F B, Sacks F, Willett W C. (2001) Dietary fats and prevention of cardiovascular disease. Patient compliance should have been considered. *British Medical Journal* **323:** 1001–2.

Hulley S, Grady D, Bush T, Furberg C, Herrington D, Riggs B, Vittinghoff E. (1998) Randomized trial of estrogen plus progestin for secondary prevention of coronary heart disease in postmenopausal women. Heart and Estrogen/progestin Replacement Study (HERS) Research Group. *Journal of the American Medical Association* **280:** 605–13.

Humphries S E, Kessling A M, Horsthemke B, Donald J A, Seed M, Jowett N, Holm M, Galton D J, Wynn V, Williamson R. (1985) A common DNA polymorphism of the low-density lipoprotein (LDL) receptor gene and its use in diagnosis. *Lancet* **i:** 1003–5.

Illingworth D R, Sexton G J. (1984) Hypocholesterolemic effects of mevinolin in patients with heterozygous familial hypercholesterolemia. *Journal of Clinical Investigation* **74:** 1972–8.

Imai H, Werthessen N T, Taylor C B, Lee K T. (1976) Angiotoxicity and arteriosclerosis due to contaminants of USP-grade cholesterol. *Archives of Pathology and Laboratory Medicine* **100:** 565–72.

Innerarity T L, Mahley R W. (1978) Enhanced binding by cultured human fibroblasts of apo-E-containing lipoproteins as compared with low density lipoproteins. *Biochemistry* **17:** 1440–7.

James A T, Martin A J. (1954) Gas-liquid chromatography; a technique for the analysis and identification of volatile materials. *British Medical Bulletin* **10:** 170–6.

James A T, Martin A J. (1956) Gas-liquid chromatography: the separation and identification of the methyl esters of saturated and unsaturated acids from formic acid to n-octadecanoic acid. *Biochemical Journal* **63:** 144–52.

Jenkins D J, Kendall C W, Marchie A, Faulkner D A, Wong J M, de Souza R, Emam A, Parker T L, Vidgen E, Trautwein E A, Lapsley K G, Josse R G, Leiter L A, Singer W, Connelly P W. (2005) Direct comparison of a dietary portfolio of cholesterol-lowering foods with a statin in hypercholesterolemic participants. *American Journal of Clinical Nutrition* **81:** 380–7.

Joslin E P. (1927) Atherosclerosis and diabetes. *Annals of Clinical Medicine* **5:** 1061–80.

Joslin E P. (1956) Diabetes for the diabetics: Ninth Banting Memorial Lecture of the British Diabetic Association. *Diabetes* **5:** 137–46.

Juhan-Vague I, Alessi M C, Mavri A, Morange P E. (2003) Plasminogen activator inhibitor-1, inflammation, obesity, insulin resistance and vascular risk. *Journal of Thrombosis and Haemostasis* **1:** 1575–9.

Julius U, Leonhardt W, Schulze J, Schollberg K, Hanefeld M, Haller H. (1981) Hyperinsulinemia in patients with low fractional catabolic rate of triglycerides. *Acta Diabetologica Latina* **18:** 217–23.

Jurgens G, Lang J, Esterbauer H. (1986) Modification of human low-density lipoprotein by the lipid peroxidation product 4-hydroxynonenal. *Biochimica et Biophysica Acta* **875:** 103–14.

Kajantie E, Osmond C, Barker D J, Forsen T, Phillips D I, Eriksson J G. (2005) Size at birth as a predictor of mortality in adulthood: a follow-up of 350 000 person-years. *International Journal of Epidemiology* **34:** 655–63.

Katan M B. (1986) Apolipoprotein E isoforms, serum cholesterol, and cancer. *Lancet* **i:** 507–8. Reprinted in the *International Journal of Epidemiology* (2004) **33:** 9.

Kay H D. (1951) The National Institute for Research in Dairying, Shinfield, Reading. *Proceedings of the Royal Society of London. Series A, Mathematical and Physical Sciences* **205:** 453–67.

Keavney B. (2004) Commentary: Katan's remarkable foresight: genes and causality 18 years on. *International Journal of Epidemiology* **33:** 11–14.

Keech A, Simes R J, Barter P, Best J, Scott R, Taskinen M R, Forder P, Pillai A, Davis T, Glasziou P, Drury P, Kesaniemi Y A, Sullivan D, Hunt D, Colman P, d'Emden M, Whiting M, Ehnholm C, Laakso M; FIELD study investigators. (2005) Effects of long-term fenofibrate therapy on cardiovascular events in 9795 people with type 2 diabetes mellitus (the FIELD study): randomized controlled trial. *Lancet* **366:** 1849–61.

Keys A. (1950) *The Biology of Human Starvation*, 2 vols. Minneapolis, MN: University of Minnesota Press. Collaborators from the Laboratory of Physiological Hygiene, School of Public Health, University of Minnesota, include: J Brozek, A Henschel, O Mickelsen, H L Taylor, E Simonson, A S Skinner, S M Wells.

Keys A. (1951) Cholesterol, 'giant molecules', and atherosclerosis. *Journal of the American Medical Association* **147:** 1514–19.

Keys A. (ed.) (1955) Arteriosclerosis: A Symposium. *Minnesota Medicine* **38:** 731–808; 829–935. Also as Keys A. (ed.) (1956) *Arteriosclerosis: A symposium presented by the Minnesota Heart Association and the University of Minnesota, 7–9 September 1955.* Minneapolis, MN: University of Minnesota Press.

Keys A. (1970) Coronary heart disease in seven countries. *Circulation* **41:** 1–211.

Keys A. (1980) *Seven Countries: A multivariate analysis of death and coronary heart disease*. London: Harvard University Press.

Keys A, Anderson J T, Grande F. (1957) Prediction of serum cholesterol responses of man to changes in fats in the diet. *Lancet* **ii:** 959–66.

Keys A, Kimura N, Kusukawa A, Bronte-Stewart B, Larsen N, Keys M H. (1958) Lessons from serum cholesterol studies in Japan, Hawaii and Los Angeles. *Annals of Internal Medicine* **48:** 83–94.

Keys A, Taylor HL, Blackburn H, Brozek J, Anderson JT, Simonson E. (1963) Coronary heart disease among Minnesota business and professional men followed 15 years. *Circulation* **28:** 381–95.

Keys A, Menotti A, Aravanis C, Blackburn H, Djordevič B S, Buzina R, Dontas A S, Fidanza F, Karvonen M J, Kimura N, Mohaček I, Nedeljkovič S, Puddu V, Punsar S, Taylor H L, Conti S, Daan Kromhout D, Toshima H. (1984) The seven countries study: 2 289 deaths in 15 years. *Preventive Medicine* **13:** 141–54.

Kinsell L W, Sinclair H M. (1957) Fats and disease. *Lancet* **272:** 883–4.

Knott T J, Rall S C Jr, Innerarity T L, Jacobson S F, Urdea M S, Levy-Wilson B, Powell L M, Pease R J, Eddy R, Nakai H, Byers M, Priestley L M, Robertson E, Rall L B, Betsholtz C, Shows T B, Mahley R W, Scott J. (1985) Human apolipoprotein B: structure of carboxyl-terminal domains, sites of gene expression, and chromosomal localization. *Science* **230:** 37–43.

Knott T J, Pease R J, Powell L M, Wallis S C, Rall S C Jr, Innerarity T L, Blackhart B, Taylor W H, Marcel Y, Milne R, Johnson D, Fuller M, Lusis A J, McCarthy B J, Mahley R W, Levy-Wilson B, Scott J. (1986) Complete protein sequence and identification of structural domains of human apolipoprotein B. *Nature* **323:** 734–8.

Kohn J. (1957) An immuno-electrophoretic technique. *Nature* **180:** 986–7.

Kohn J. (1970) Electrophoresis and immunodiffusion techniques on cellulose acetate membrane. *Methods in Medical Research* **12:** 243–60.

Krieger M. (1992) Molecular flypaper and atherosclerosis: structure of the macrophage scavenger receptor. *Trends in Biochemical Sciences* **17:** 141–6.

Kyle R A, Shampo M A. (1997) Theodor Svedberg and the ultracentrifuge. *Mayo Clinic Proceedings* **72:** 830.

Laakso M. (1995) Epidemiology of diabetic dyslipidaemia. *Diabetic Review* **3:** 408–22.

Langer T, Strober W, Levy R I. (1972) The metabolism of low density lipoprotein in familial type II hyperlipoproteinemia. *Journal of Clinical Investigation* **51:** 1528–36.

Law M. (2000) Plant sterol and stanol margarines and health. *British Medical Journal* **320:** 861–4.

Lawlor D A, Ebrahim S, Davey Smith G. (2001) Sex matters: secular and geographical trends in sex differences in coronary heart disease mortality. *British Medical Journal* **323:** 541–5. Erratum in *BMJ* (2002) **325:** 580.

Lendon C, Born G V R, Davies M J, Richardson P D. (1992) Plaque fissure: the link between atherosclerosis and thrombosis. *Nouvelle revue Francaise d'hematologie* **34:** 27–9.

Lendrum A C. (1949) The staining of erythrocytes in tissue sections a new method and observations on some of the modified mallory connective tissue stains. *Journal of Pathology and Bacteriology* **61:** 443–8.

Leren P. (1970) The Oslo diet–heart study. Eleven-year report. *Circulation* **42:** 935–42.

Levy R I, Langer T. (1971) Hypolipidemic drugs and hyperlipoproteinemia. *Annals of the New York Academy of Sciences* **179:** 475–80.

Lewis S M, Collier I C. (1992) Appendix B: Laboratory Values. In Ladig D J, Van Schaik T. *Medical Surgical Nursing, Assessment and Management of Clinical Problems*. 3rd edn. St Louis, MO: Mosby-Year Book Inc.

Lewis T. (1932) The relation of clinical medicine to physiology from the standpoint of research. *British Medical Journal* **ii:** 1046–9.

Lewis T. (1946) *Diseases of the Heart: Described for practitioners and students.* 4th edn. London: Macmillan.

Lipid Research Clinics (LRC) Coronary Primary Prevention Trial. (1984) The Lipid Research Clinics Coronary Primary Prevention Trial results. I. Reduction in incidence of coronary heart disease; II. The relationship of reduction in incidence of coronary heart disease to cholesterol lowering. *Journal of the American Medical Association* **251:** 351–64; 365–74.

Logan W P D, Morris J N. (1952) Letter to the Editor: cooperation in research on heart disease. *Lancet* **i:** 1116.

Long-Term Intervention with Pravastatin in Ischemic Disease (LIPID) Study Group. (1988) Prevention of cardiovascular events and death with pravastatin in patients with coronary heart disease and a broad range of initial cholesterol levels. *New England Journal of Medicine* **339:** 1349–57.

Long-Term Intervention with Pravastatin in Ischemic Disease (LIPID) Study. (1995) Design features and baseline characteristics of the LIPID (Long-Term Intervention with Pravastatin in Ischemic Disease) Study: a randomized trial in patients with previous acute myocardial infarction and/or unstable angina pectoris. *American Journal of Cardiology* **76:** 474–9.

Lovastatin Study Group II. (1986) Therapeutic response to lovastatin (mevinolin) in nonfamilial hypercholesterolemia. A multicenter study. *Journal of the American Medical Association* **256:** 2829–34.

Lovastatin Study Group III. (1988) A multicenter comparison of lovastatin and cholestyramine therapy for severe primary hypercholesterolemia. *Journal of the American Medical Association* **260:** 359–66.

Lovastatin Study Group IV. (1990). A multicenter comparison of lovastatin and probucol for treatment of severe primary hypercholesterolemia. *American Journal of Cardiology* **66:** 22b–30b.

Lowe G D, McArdle B M, Stromberg P, Lorimer A R, Forbes C D, Prentice C R. (1982) Increased blood viscosity and fibrinolytic inhibitor in type II hyperlipoproteinaemia. *Lancet* **i:** 472–5.

Lowe G D, Drummond M M, Third J L, Bremner W F, Forbes C D, Prentice C R, Lawrie T D. (1980) Increased plasma fibrinogen and platelet-aggregates in type II hyperlipoproteinaemia. *Thrombosis and Haemostasis* **42:** 1503–7.

Lowe G D, Wood D A, Douglas J T, Riemersma R A, Macintyre C C, Takase T, Tuddenham E G, Forbes C D, Elton R A, Oliver M F. (1991) Relationships of plasma viscosity, coagulation and fibrinolysis to coronary risk factors and angina. *Thrombosis and Haemostasis* **65:** 339–43.

Mabuchi H, Haba T, Tatami R, Miyamoto S, Sakai Y, Wakasugi T, Watanabe A, Koizumi J, Takeda R. (1981) Effect of an inhibitor of 3-hydroxy-3-methyglutaryl coenzyme A reductase on serum lipoproteins and ubiquinone-10-levels in patients with familial hypercholesterolemia. *New England Journal of Medicine* **305:** 478–82.

MacCallum P K, Rudnicka A R, Rumley A, Meade T W, Lowe G D. (2004) Low-intensity warfarin reduces thrombin generation and fibrin turnover, but not low-grade inflammation, in men at risk of myocardial infarction. *British Journal of Haematology* **127:** 448–50.

Mahley R W, Innerarity T L. (1978) Properties of lipoproteins responsible for high affinity binding to cell surface receptors of fibroblasts and smooth muscle cells. In Kritchevsky D, Paoletti R, Holmes W L. (eds) *Drugs, Lipid Metabolism and Atherosclerosis.* New York, NY: Plenum Publishing Corporation, 99–127.

Mann J, Skeaff M, Truswell S. (2001) Dietary fats and prevention of cardiovascular disease. Conclusion may have been underplayed. *British Medical Journal* **323:** 1000–1; author reply 1001–2.

Marmot M G, Rose G, Shipley M, Hamilton P J. (1978) Employment grade and coronary heart disease in British civil servants. *Journal of Epidemiology and Community Health* **32:** 244–9.

Martin A J, James A T. (1956) Gas–liquid chromatography: the gas-density meter, a new apparatus for the detection of vapours in flowing gas streams. *Biochemical Journal* **63:** 138–43.

McCord J M, Fridovich I. (1969) Superoxide dismutase. An enzymic function for erythrocuprein (hemocuprein). *Journal of Biological Chemistry* **244:** 6049–55.

McKeigue P M, Marmot M G, Adelstein A M, Hunt S P, Shipley M J, Butler S M, Riemersma R A, Turner P R. (1985) Diet and risk factors for coronary heart disease in Asians in northwest London. *Lancet* **ii:** 1086–90.

McMichael J. (1979) Fats and atheroma: an inquest. *British Medical Journal* **i:** 173–5.

McNicol G P, Douglas A S. (1964) Epsilon-aminocaproic acid and other inhibitors of fibrinolysis. *British Medical Bulletin* **20:** 233–9.

Meade T W, Ruddock V, Stirling Y, Chakrabarti R, Miller G J. (1993) Fibrinolytic activity, clotting factors, and long-term incidence of ischaemic heart disease in the Northwick Park Heart Study. *Lancet* **342:** 1076–9.

Medical Research Council's General Practice Research Framework. (1998) Thrombosis prevention trial: randomized trial of low-intensity oral anticoagulation with warfarin and low-dose aspirin in the primary prevention of ischaemic heart disease in men at increased risk. *Lancet* **351:** 233–41.

Mensink R P, Katan M B. (1992) Effect of dietary fatty acids on serum lipids and lipoproteins. A meta-analysis of 27 trials. *Arteriosclerosis and Thrombosis* **12:** 911–19.

Miller G J. (1999) Lipoproteins and the haemostatic system in atherothrombotic disorders. *Bailliere's Best Practice and Research: Clinical Haematology* **12:** 555–75.

Miller G J, Miller N E. (1975) Plasma-high-density-lipoprotein (HDL) concentration and development of ischaemic heart disease. *Lancet* **i:** 16–19.

Miller G J, Walter S J, Stirling Y, Thompson S G, Esnouf M P, Meade T W. (1985) Assay of factor VII activity by two techniques: evidence for increased conversion of VII to alpha VIIa in hyperlipidaemia, with possible implications for ischaemic heart disease. *British Journal of Haematology* **59:** 249–58.

Mitchell J R A. (1984) What constitutes evidence on the dietary prevention of coronary heart disease? Cosy beliefs or harsh facts? *International Journal of Cardiology* **5:** 287–98.

Mitchell J R A. (1985) Diet and arterial disease: the myths and the realities. *Proceedings of the Nutrition Society* **44:** 363–70.

Mitchell J R A, for GRAND (Glaxo Receptor Antagonist against Nottingham DVT) Study Group. (1987) *Trial of Thromboxane Receptor Antagonist as Prophylaxis Against Deep Vein Thrombosis in Suspected Acute Myocardial Infarction*. Uxbridge, Middlesex: Glaxo [Glaxo internal report].

Mitchell J R A, Schwartz C J. (1965) *Arterial Disease*. Oxford: Blackwell Scientific Publications.

Morgagni G B. (1762) *De sedibus, et causis morborum per anatomen indagatis, libri quinque*. Naples: Simoni [vols. II-III, Raymundi for D. Terres].

Morris J N. (1951) Recent history of coronary disease. *Lancet* **i:** 1–7; 69–73.

Morris J N. (1957) *Uses of Epidemiology*. Edinburgh; London: E & S Livingstone.

Morris J N. (1960) Occupation and coronary heart disease. In Medical Research Council, *Current Medical Research*. London: HMSO, 1–4.

Morris J N, Crawford M D. (1958) Coronary heart disease and physical activity of work; evidence of a national necropsy survey. *British Medical Journal* **ii:** 1485–96.

Morris J N, Dale R A. (1955) Epidemiology of coronary atherosclerosis. *Proceedings of the Royal Society of Medicine* **48:** 667–73.

Morris J N, Raffle P A B. (1954) Coronary heart disease in transport workers: a progress report. *British Journal of Industrial Medicine* **11:** 260–4.

Morris J N, Heady J A, Barley R G. (1952) Coronary heart disease in medical practitioners. *British Medical Journal* **i:** 503–20.

Morris J N, Heady J A, Raffle P A, Roberts C G, Parks J W. (1953) Coronary heart-disease and physical activity of work. *Lancet* **265:** 1053–7; 1111–20.

Morris J N, Everitt M G, Pollard R, Chave S P, Semmence A M. (1980) Vigorous exercise in leisure-time: protection against coronary heart disease. *Lancet* **ii:** 1207–10.

Morris J N, Chave S P, Adam C, Sirey C, Epstein L, Sheehan D J. (1973) Vigorous exercise in leisure-time and the incidence of coronary heart disease. *Lancet* **i:** 333–9.

Moschcowitz E. (1942) *Vascular Sclerosis with special reference to arteriosclerosis.* New York, NY: Oxford University Press.

Müller C. (1939) Angina pectoris in hereditary xanthomatosis. *Archives of Internal Medicine* **64:** 675–700.

Mullis K B. (1990) The unusual origin of the polymerase chain reaction. *Scientific American* **262:** 56–65.

Mullis K B, Faloona F, Scharf S, Saiki R, Horn G, Erlich H. (1986) Specific enzymatic amplification of DNA *in vitro*: the polymerase chain reaction. *Cold Spring Harbor Symposia on Quantitative Biology* **51:** 263–73.

Multicentre Anti-Atheroma Study (MAAS). (1994) Effect of simvastatin on coronary atheroma: the Multicentre Anti-Atheroma Study (MAAS). *Lancet* **344:** 633–8. Erratum in *Lancet* **344:** 762.

Multiple Risk Factor Intervention Trial (MRFIT). (1976) The multiple risk factor intervention trial (MRFIT). A national study of primary prevention of coronary heart disease. *Journal of the American Medical Association* **235:** 825–7.

Multiple Risk Factor Intervention Trial Research Group (1982) Multiple risk factor intervention trial. Risk factor changes and mortality results. *Journal of the American Medical Association* **248:** 1465–77.

Myant N B. (1990a) *Cholesterol Metabolism, LDL and the LDL Receptor.* San Diego, CA; London: Academic Press.

Myant N B. (1990b) Current approaches to the genetics of coronary heart disease (CHD) including an account of work done at Hammersmith Hospital. *Bollettino della Societa Italiana di Biologia Sperimentale* **66:** 1015–41.

Myant N B. (1993) Familial defective apolipoprotein B-100: a review, including some comparisons with familial hypercholesterolaemia. *Atherosclerosis* **104:** 1–18.

Neroth P. (2005) Interview: Advice from the heart. *New Scientist* **185**(2486): 44–7. Freely available at www.newscientist.com/channel/opinion/mg18524861.700.html (visited 21 November 2005).

Ness A R, Reynolds L A, Tansey E M. (eds) (2002) Population-based Research in South Wales: The MRC Pneumoconiosis Research Unit and the MRC Epidemiology Unit. *Wellcome Witnesses to Twentieth Century Medicine*, vol. 13. London: The Wellcome Trust Centre for the History of Medicine at UCL. Freely available from www.ucl.ac.uk/histmed following links to Publications/Wellcome Witnesses.

Nevin N C, Slack J. (1968) Hyperlipidaemic xanthomatosis: II. Mode of inheritance in 55 families with essential hyperlipidaemia and xanthomatosis. *Journal of Medical Genetics* **5:** 9–28.

New M I, Roberts T N, Bierman E L, Reader G G. (1963) The significance of blood lipid alterations in diabetes mellitus. *Diabetes* **12:** 208–12.

Nikkilä E A. (1953) Studies on the lipid-protein relationship in normal and pathological sera and the effect of heparin on serum lipoproteins. *Scandinavian Journal of Clinical and Laboratory Investigation* **5:** 9–100.

Nikkilä E A, Hormila P. (1978) Serum lipids and lipoproteins in insulin-treated diabetes. Demonstration of increased high-density lipoprotein concentrations. *Diabetes* **27:** 1078–86.

Oliver M F. (1962a) Reduction of serum lipid and uric acid levels by an orally active androsterone. *Lancet* **i:** 1321–3.

Oliver M F. (1962b) Further observations of the effects of *Atromid* and of ethylchlorophenoxyisobutyrate on serum lipid levels. *Journal of Atherosclerosis Research* **3:** 427–44.

Oliver M F, Boyd G S. (1953a) Changes in the plasma lipids during the menstrual cycle. *Clinical Science* **12:** 217–22.

Oliver M F, Boyd G S. (1953b) The clearing by heparin of alimentary lipaemia in coronary artery disease. *Clinical Science* **12:** 293–8.

Oliver M F, Boyd G S. (1953c) The plasma lipids in coronary artery disease. *British Heart Journal* **15:** 387–92. The communication to the British Cardiac Society was published on page 466, the full article appears in the same volume.

Oliver M F, Boyd G S. (1955) Serum lipoprotein patterns in coronary sclerosis and associated conditions. *British Heart Journal* **17:** 299–302.

Oliver M F, Boyd G S. (1961) Influence of reduction of serum lipids on prognosis of coronary artery disease – a five-year study using oestrogen. *Lancet* **ii:** 499–505.

Osler W. (1910) Lumleian Lecture: angina pectoris. *Lancet* **i:** 697–702.

Padley F B, Timms R E. (1978) Determination of cocoa butter equivalents in chocolate. *Chemistry and industry* **(23):** 918–19.

Paneth N, Susser M. (1995) Editorial: Early origin of coronary heart disease (the 'Barker hypothesis'). *British Medical Journal* **310:** 411–12.

Patterson D, Slack J. (1972) Lipid abnormalities in male and female survivors of myocardial infarction and their first-degree relatives. *Lancet* **i:** 393–9.

Pietinen P, Aro A, Tuomilehto J, Uusitalo U, Korhonen H. (1990) Consumption of boiled coffee is correlated with serum cholesterol in Finland. *International Journal of Epidemiology* **19**: 586–90.

Pitas R E, Innerarity T L, Arnold K S, Mahley R W. (1979) Rate and equilibrium constants for binding of apo-E HDLc (a cholesterol-induced lipoprotein) and low density lipoproteins to human fibroblasts: evidence for multiple receptor binding of apo-E HDLc. *Proceedings of the National Academy of Sciences of the USA* **76:** 2311–15.

Pooling Project Research Group. (1978) Relationship of blood pressure, serum cholesterol, smoking habit, relative weight and ECG abnormalities to incidence of major coronary events: final report of the pooling project. *Journal of Chronic Diseases* **31:** 201–306.

Popják G. (1958) Biosynthesis of cholesterol. *British Medicial Bulletin* **14:** 221–6.

Powell L M, Wallis S C, Pease R J, Edwards Y H, Knott T J, Scott J. (1987) A novel form of tissue-specific RNA processing produces apolipoprotein-B48 in intestine. *Cell* **50:** 831–40.

Price F W. (1950) *A Textbook of the Practice of Medicine*. 8th edn. Oxford Medical Publications series. London: Oxford University Press.

Principal Investigators. (1978) A cooperative trial in the primary prevention of ischaemic heart disease using clofibrate. Report of the Committee of Principal Investigators. *British Heart Journal* **40:** 1069–118.

Principal Investigators. (1984) WHO cooperative trial on primary prevention of ischaemic heart disease with clofibrate to lower serum cholesterol: final mortality follow-up. Report of the Committee of Principal Investigators. *Lancet* **ii:** 600–4.

Prospective Pravastatin Pooling (PPP) project. (1995) Design, rational, and baseline characteristics of the Prospective Pravastatin Pooling (PPP) project – a combined analysis of three large-scale randomized trials: Long-term Intervention with Pravastatin in Ischemic Disease (LIPID), Cholesterol and Recurrent Events (CARE), and West of Scotland Coronary Prevention Study (WOSCOPS). *American Journal of Cardiology* **76:** 899–905.

Puska P, Tuomilehto J, Salonen J, Nissinen A, Koskela K, Vartiainen E, *et al.* (1981) *Community Control of Cardiovascular Disease: Evaluation of a comprehensive community programme for control of cardiovascular diseases in North Karelia, Finland, 1972–77*. Copenhagen: World Health Organization, Regional Office for Europe, for the National Public Health Laboratory of Finland.

Randle P J, Bell J, Scott J. (eds) (1990) *Genetics and Human Nutrition:* International symposium papers. London: John Libbey.

Raz I, Havivi Y, Yarom R. (1998) Reduced negative surface charge on arterial endothelium of diabetic rats. *Diabetologia* **31:** 618–20.

Reaven G M. (1988) Banting Lecture 1988: Role of insulin resistance in human disease. *Diabetes* **37:** 1595–607.

Reckless J P, Galton D J. (1980) Peripheral resistance to the cellular action of insulin in obese diabetic subjects *in vivo. Clinical Science* **58:** 59–63.

Reckless J P, Betteridge D J, Wu P, Payne B, Galton D J. (1978) High-density and low-density lipoproteins and prevalence of vascular disease in diabetes mellitus. *British Medical Journal* **i:** 883–6.

Rees A, Shoulders C C, Stocks J, Galton D J, Baralle F E. (1983) DNA polymorphism adjacent to human apoprotein A-1 gene: relation to hypertriglyceridaemia. *Lancet* **i:** 444–6.

Rees A, Stocks J, Sharpe C R, Vella M A, Shoulders C C, Katz J, Jowett N I, Baralle F E, Galton D J. (1985) Deoxyribonucleic acid polymorphism in the apolipoprotein A-1-C-III gene cluster. Association with hypertriglyceridemia. *Journal of Clinical Investigation* **76:** 1090–5.

Reynolds L A, Tansey E M. (eds) (2000) Clinical Research in Britain, 1950–80. *Wellcome Witnesses to Twentieth Century Medicine*, vol. 7. London: The Wellcome Trust. Freely available online at www.ucl.ac.uk/histmed following the links to Publications/Wellcome Witnesses.

Reynolds L A, Tansey E M. (eds) (2005) The Recent History of Platelets in Thrombosis and Other Disorders. *Wellcome Witnesses to Twentieth Century Medicine*, vol. 23. London: The Wellcome Trust Centre for the History of Medicine at UCL. Freely available online at www.ucl.ac.uk/histmed following the links to Publications/Wellcome Witnesses.

Richardson P D, Davies M J, Born G V R. (1989) Influence of plaque configuration and stress distribution on fissuring of coronary atherosclerotic plaques. *Lancet* **ii:** 941–4.

Richmond W. (1973) Preparation and properties of a cholesterol oxidase from *Nocardia* sp. and its application to the enzymatic assay of total cholesterol in serum. *Clinical Chemistry* **19:** 1350–6.

Richmond W. (1974) Proceedings: The development of an enzymic technique for the assay of cholesterol in biological fluids. *Clinical Science and Molecular Medicine* **46:** 6P–7P.

Richmond W. (1976) Use of cholesterol oxidase for assay of total and free cholesterol in serum by continuous-flow analysis. *Clinical Chemistry* **22:** 1579–88.

Rifkind B M, Segal P. (1983) Lipid Research Clinics Program reference values for hyperlipidemia and hypolipidemia. *Journal of the American Medical Association* **250:** 1869–72.

Robertson F W, Cumming A M. (1985) Effects of apoprotein E polymorphism on serum lipoprotein concentration. *Arteriosclerosis* **5:** 283–92.

Robertson G, Cramp D G. (1970) An evaluation of cholesterol determinations in serum and serum lipoprotein fractions by a semi-automated fluorimetric method. *Journal of Clinical Pathology* **23:** 243–5.

Rose G A. (1964) Familial patterns in ischaemic heart disease. *British Journal of Preventive and Social Medicine* **18:** 75–80.

Rose G A. (1981) Strategy of prevention: lessons from cardiovascular disease. *British Medical Journal* **282:** 1847–51.

Rose G A, Heller R F, Pedoe H T, Christie D G. (1980) Heart disease prevention project: a randomized controlled trial in industry. *British Medical Journal* **280:** 747–51.

Rose G A, Blackburn H, Keys A, Taylor H L, Kannel W B, Paul O, Reid D D, Stamler J. (1974) Colon cancer and blood-cholesterol. *Lancet* **i:** 181–3.

Royal College of Physicians of London and the British Cardiac Society. (1976) *Prevention of Coronary Heart Disease: Report of a Joint Working Party.* London: Royal College of Physicians of London. Dr A G Shaper, Chairman. Originally published in the *Journal of the Royal College of Physicians* (1975) **10:** 213–75.

Royal Pharmaceutical Society, practice division. (2004) Practice guidance: OTC simvastatin 10mg. *Pharmaceutical Journal* **273:** 169–70.

Rubins H B, Robins S J, Collins D, Fye C L, Anderson J W, Elam M B, Faas F H, Linares E, Schaefer E J, Schectman G, Wilt T J, Wittes J, for the Veterans Affairs High-Density Lipoprotein Cholesterol Intervention Trial Study Group. (1999) Gemfibrozil for the secondary prevention of coronary heart disease in men with low levels of high-density lipoprotein cholesterol. *New England Journal of Medicine* **341:** 410–18.

Ryle J A, Russell W T. (1949) The natural history of coronary disease. *British Heart Journal* **11:** 370–8.

Sacks F M, Pfeffer M A, Moye L A, Brown L E, Hamm P, Cole T G, Hawkins C M, Braunwald E. (1992) Rationale and design of a secondary prevention trial of lowering normal plasma cholesterol levels after acute myocardial infarction: the Cholesterol and Recurrent Events trial (CARE). *American Journal of Cardiology* **68:** 1436–46. Erratum in *American Journal of Cardiology* **69**: 574.

Sacks F M, Pfeffer M A, Moye L A, Rouleau J L, Rutherford J D, Cole T G, Brown L E, Warnica J W, Arnold J M, Wun C C, Davis B R, Braunwald E. (1996) The effect of pravastatin on coronary events after myocardial infarction in patients with average cholesterol levels. Cholesterol and Recurrent Events Trial investigators. *New England Journal of Medicine* **335:** 1001–9.

Sanders T A B. (1987) Diet and coronary heart disease. *Journal of the Royal Society of Health* **107:** 163–5.

Sanders T A B. (1988) Dietary fat and coronary heart disease. In Dobbing J. (ed.) *A Balanced Diet.* Berlin, Heidelberg: Springer-Verlag, 993–1116.

Sanders T A B. (2001) A life of good taste. *Nature* **413:** 360–1.

Sanders T A B, Ellis F R, Dickerson J W. (1978) Studies of vegans: the fatty acid composition of plasma choline phosphoglycerides, erythrocytes, adipose tissue, and breast milk, and some indicators of susceptibility to ischemic heart disease in vegans and omnivore controls. *American Journal of Clinical Nutrition* **31:** 805–13.

Scandinavian Simvastatin Survival Study (4S). (1993) Design and baseline results of the Scandinavian Simvastatin Survival Study of patients with stable angina and/or previous myocardial infarction. *American Journal of Cardiology* **71:** 393–400.

Scandinavian Simvastatin Survival Study (4S). (1994) Randomized trial of cholesterol lowering in 4444 patients with coronary heart disease. *Lancet* **344:** 1383–9.

Schaffner C P, Gordon H W. (1968) The hypocholesterolemic activity of orally-administered polyene macrolides. *Proceedings of the National Academy of Sciences of the USA* **61:** 36–41.

Segrest J P, Jackson R L, Morrisett J D, Gotto A M Jr. (1974) A molecular theory of lipid-protein interactions in the plasma lipoproteins. *FEBS Letters* **38:** 247–58.

Shaper A G. (1962) Cardiovascular studies in the Samburu tribe of Northern Kenya. *American Heart Journal* **63:** 437–42.

Shaper A G. (1972) Diet in the epidemiology of coronary heart disease. Proceedings of the *Nutrition Society* **31:** 297–302.

Shaper A G, Jones K W, Jones M, Kyobe J. (1963) Serum lipids in three nomadic tribes of northern Kenya. *American Journal of Clinical Nutrition* **13:** 135–46.

Shaper A G, Jones K W, Kyobe J, Jones M. (1966) Fibrinolysis in relation to body fatness, serum lipids and coronary heart disease in African and Asian men in Uganda. *Journal of Atherosclerosis Research* **6:** 313–27.

Shepherd J, Bicker S, Lorimer A R, Packard C J. (1979) Receptor-mediated low-density lipoprotein catabolism in man. *Journal of Lipid Research* **20:** 999–1006.

Shepherd J, Cobbe S M, Ford I, Isles C G, Lorimer A R, MacFarlane P W, McKillop J H, Packard C J. (1995) Prevention of coronary heart disease with pravastatin in men with hypercholesterolemia. West of Scotland Coronary Prevention Study Group. *New England Journal of Medicine* **333:** 1301–7.

Shepherd J, Blauw G J, Murphy M B, Cobbe S M, Bollen E L, Buckley B M, Ford I, Jukema J W, Hyland M, Gaw A, Lagaay A M, Perry I J, Macfarlane P W, Meinders A E, Sweeney B J, Packard C J, Westendorp R G, Twomey C, Stott D J. (1999) The design of a prospective study of Pravastatin in the Elderly at Risk (PROSPER). PROSPER Study Group. *American Journal of Cardiology* **84:** 1192–7.

Shoulders C C, Baralle F E. (1982) Isolation of the human HDL apoprotein A1 gene. *Nucleic Acids Research* **10:** 4873–82.

Simionescu M. (1980) Structural and functional differentiation of microvascular endothelium. *Ciba Foundation Symposium* **71:** 39–60.

Simpson H C, Simpson R W, Lousley S, Carter R D, Geekie M, Hockaday T D, Mann J I. (1981) A high carbohydrate leguminous fibre diet improves all aspects of diabetic control. *Lancet* **i:** 1–5.

Sinclair H M. (1956) Deficiency of essential fatty acids and atherosclerosis etcetera. *Lancet* **i:** 381–3.

Sing C F, Davignon J. (1985) Role of the apolipoprotein E polymorphism in determining normal plasma lipid and lipoprotein variation. *American Journal of Human Genetics* **37:** 268–85.

Siperstein M D, Fagan V M. (1964) Studies on the feedback regulation of cholesterol synthesis. *Advances in Enzyme Regulation* **2:** 249–64.

Slack J. (1969) Risks of ischaemic heart disease in familial hyperlipoproteinaemic states. *Lancet* **ii:** 1380–2.

Slack J, Evans K A. (1966) The increased risk of death from ischaemic heart disease in first degree relatives of 121 men and 96 women with ischaemic heart disease. *Journal of Medical Genetics* **3:** 239–57.

Slack J, Nevin N C. (1968) Hyperlipidaemic xanthomatosis: I. Increased risk of death from ischaemic heart disease in first degree relatives of 53 patients with essential hyperlipidaemia and xanthomatosis. *Journal of Medical Genetics* **5:** 4–8.

Smith E B. (1965) The influence of age and atherosclerosis on the chemistry of aortic intima. 1. The lipids. *Journal of Atherosclerosis Research* **5:** 224–40.

Smith E B, Ashall C. (1983) Low-density lipoprotein concentration in interstitial fluid from human atherosclerotic lesions. Relation to theories of endothelial damage and lipoprotein binding. *Biochimica et Biophysica Acta* **754:** 249–57.

Smith E B, Slater R S. (1972) Relationship between low-density lipoprotein in aortic intima and serum-lipid levels. *Lancet* **i:** 463–9.

Smith E B, Staples E M. (1980) Distribution of plasma proteins across the human aortic wall – barrier functions of endothelium and internal elastic lamina. *Atherosclerosis* **37:** 579–90.

Smith E B, Staples E M. (1982) Plasma protein concentrations in interstitial fluid from human aortas. *Proceedings of the Royal Society of London, Series B, Biological Sciences* **217:** 59–75.

Smith E B, Evans P H, Downham M D. (1967) Lipid in the aortic intima. The correlation of morphological and chemical characteristics. *Journal of Atherosclerosis Research* **7:** 171–86.

Smith L C, Pownall H J, Gotto AM Jr. (1978) The plasma lipoproteins: structure and metabolism. *Annual Review of Biochemistry* **47:** 751–7.

Soutar A K, Myant N B, Thompson G R. (1977) Simultaneous measurement of apolipoprotein B turnover in very-low-and low-density lipoproteins in familial hypercholesterolaemia. *Atherosclerosis* **28:** 247–56.

Southern E M. (1975) Detection of specific sequences among DNA fragments separated by gel electrophoresis. *Journal of Molecular Biology* **98:** 503–17. Reprinted in *Biotechnology* (1992) **24:** 122–39.

Steel F. (2005) A source of our wealth, yet adverse to our health? Butter and the diet–heart link in New Zealand. *Social History of Medicine* **18:** 475–93.

Stein O, Stein Y, Eisenberg S. (1973) A radioautograph study of the transport of ^{125}I-labelled serum glycoproteins in rat aorta. *Zeitschrift fur Zellforschung und mikroskopische Anatomie* **138:** 223–37.

Steinberg D. (2004) Thematic review series: the pathogenesis of atherosclerosis. An interpretive history of the cholesterol controversy, part I. *Journal of Lipid Research* **45:** 1583–93.

Steinberg D. (2005a) The pathogenesis of atherosclerosis, part II: the early evidence linking hypercholesterolemia to coronary disease in humans. *Journal of Lipid Research* **46:** 179–90.

Steinberg D. (2005b) The pathogenesis of atherosclerosis, part III: mechanistically defining the role of hyperlipidemia. *Journal of Lipid Research* **46:** 2037–51.

Steinberg D. (2006) The pathogenesis of atherosclerosis, part IV: the 1984 coronary primary prevention trial ends it – almost. *Journal of Lipid Research* **47:** 1–14.

Strandberg T E, Pyörälä K, Cook T J, Wilhelmsen L, Faergeman O, Thorgeirsson G, Pedersen T R, Kjekshus J (4S Group). (2004) Mortality and incidence of cancer during 10-year follow-up of the Scandinavian Simvastatin Survival Study (4S). *Lancet* **364:** 771–7.

van Stuyvenberg J H. (1969) *Margarine: An economic, social and scientific history, 1869–1969.* Liverpool: Liverpool University Press.

Swales J D. (ed.) (1985) *Platt versus Pickering: An episode in recent medical history.* London: Keynes Press for the British Medical Association.

Tang J L, Armitage J M, Lancaster T, Silagy C A, Fowler G H, Neil H A. (1998) Systematic review of dietary intervention trials to lower blood total cholesterol in free-living subjects. *British Medical Journal* **316:** 1213–20.

Tansey E M, Catterall P P. (1997) Technology Transfer in Britain: The case of Monoclonal Antibodies. In Tansey E M, Catterall P P, Christie D A, Willhoft S V, Reynolds L A. (eds) (1997) *Wellcome Witnesses to Twentieth Century Medicine*, vol. 1. London: The Wellcome Trust, 1–34. Freely available online at www.ucl.ac.uk/histmed following the links to Publications/Wellcome Witnesses.

Tansey E M, Christie D A. (eds) (1999) Haemophilia: Recent history of clinical management. *Wellcome Witnesses to Twentieth Century Medicine*, vol. 4. London: The Wellcome Trust. Freely available online at www.ucl.ac.uk/histmed following the links to Publications/Wellcome Witnesses.

Tansey E M, Reynolds L A. (1997) The Committee on Safety of Drugs. In Tansey E M, Catterall P P, Christie D A, Willhoft S V, Reynolds L A. (eds) (1997) *Wellcome Witnesses to Twentieth Century Medicine*, vol. 1. London: The Wellcome Trust, 103–35. Freely available online at www.ucl.ac.uk/histmed following the links to Publications/Wellcome Witnesses.

Thannhauser S J. (1940) *Lipoidoses.* New York, NY: Oxford University Press.

Thannhauser S J. (1950) *Lipoidoses: Diseases of the cellular lipid metabolism.* 2nd edn. New York, NY: Oxford University Press.

Thompson G R. (1974) Beware sweet reason in the search for causes of heart disease. *The Times* (31 July): 16.

Thompson G R. (1983) Plasma exchange and affinity chromatographic therapy for hyperlipidaemia: a review. *Apheresis Bulletin* **1:** 26–31.

Thompson G R. (1999) *Hammersmith Marathon.* London: Royal Society of Medicine Press.

Thompson G R, Lewis B, Booth C C. (1966) Absorption of vitamin D3-3H in control subjects and patients with intestinal malabsorption. *Journal of Clinical Investigation* **45:** 94–102.

Thompson G R, Lowenthal R, Myant N B. (1975) Plasma exchange in the management of homozygous familial hypercholesterolaemia. *Lancet* **i:** 1208–11.

Thompson G R, Miller J P, Breslow J L. (1985) Improved survival of patients with homozygous familial hypercholesterolaemia treated with plasma exchange. *British Medical Journal* **291:** 1671–3.

Thompson G R, Ford J, Jenkinson M, Trayner I. (1986) Efficacy of mevinolin as adjuvant therapy for refractory familial hypercholesterolaemia. *Quarterly Journal of Medicine* **60:** 803–11.

Thompson G R, Myant N B, Kilpatrick D, Oakley C M, Raphael M J, Steiner R E. (1980) Assessment of long-term plasma exchange for familial hypercholesterolaemia. *British Heart Journal* **43:** 680–8.

Thomson A L. (1975, 1987) *Half a Century of Medical Research: vol. 2. The programme of the Medical Research Council (UK)*. London: Medical Research Council.

Thorp J M, Waring W S. (1962) Modification of metabolism and distribution of lipids by ethyl chlorophenoxyisobutyrate. *Nature* **194:** 948–9.

Tobert J A. (1987) New developments in lipid-lowering therapy: the role of inhibitors of hydroxymethylglutaryl-coenzyme A reductase. *Circulation* **76:** 534–8.

Tobert J A. (2003) Lovastatin and beyond: the history of the HMG-CoA reductase inhibitors. *Nature Reviews-Drug Discovery* **2:** 517–26.

Tobert J A, Hitzenberger G, Kukovetz W R, Holmes I B, Jones K H. (1982a) Rapid and substantial lowering of human serum cholesterol by mevinolin (MK-803), an inhibitor of hydroxymethylglutaryl-coenzyme A reductase. *Atherosclerosis* **41:** 61–5.

Tobert J A, Bell G D, Birtwell J, James I, Kukovetz W R, Pryor J S, Buntinx A, Holmes I B, Chao Y S, Bolognese J A. (1982b) Cholesterol-lowering effect of mevinolin, an inhibitor of 3-hydroxy-3-methylglutaryl-coenzyme A reductase, in healthy volunteers. *Journal of Clinical Investigation* **69:** 913–19.

Truswell A S. (1984) Editorial: end of static decade for coronary disease? *British Medical Journal* **289:** 509–10.

Tunstall-Pedoe H. (1975) Proceedings: Myocardial infarction in east London. *British Heart Journal* **37:** 550–1.

Tunstall-Pedoe H. (1978) Uses of coronary heart attack registers. *British Heart Journal* **40:** 510–15.

Tunstall-Pedoe H. (1980) Decline in mortality from coronary heart disease in America. *Lancet* **i:** 831.

Tunstall-Pedoe H, Clayton D, Morris J N, Brigden W, McDonald L. (1975) Coronary heart attacks in east London. *Lancet* **ii:** 833–8.

Tunstall-Pedoe H. (ed.) (2003) *MONICA* [MONItoring of trends and determinants in CArdiovascular disease] *Monograph and Multimedia Sourcebook. World's Largest Study of Heart Disease, Stroke, Risk Factors and Population Trends 1979–2003*. Geneva: World Health Organization.

Turnberg L A, Mahoney M P, Gleeson M H, Freeman C B, Gowenlock A H. (1972) Plasmaphoresis and plasma exchange in the treatment of hyperlipaemia and xanthomatous neuropathy in patients with primary biliary cirrhosis. *Gut* **13:** 976–81.

Turnbull H M. (1915) Alterations in arterial structure and their relation to syphilis. *Quarterly Journal of Medicine* **8:** 201–54.

Turnbull H M. (1920) *Report to the Salvarsan Committee.* I. Results of the examination of tissues from eight cases of death following injections of salvarsan. Special report series no. 55. London: HMSO.

UK Prospective Diabetes Study (UKPDS). (1991) VIII. Study design, progress and performance. *Diabetologia* **34:** 877–90.

Upritchard J E, Zeelenberg M J, Huizinga H, Verschuren P M, Trautwein E A. (2005) Modern fat technology: what is the potential for heart health? *Proceedings of the Nutrition Society* **64:** 379–86.

Utermann G, Jaeschke M, Menzel J. (1975) Familial hyperlipoproteinemia type III: deficiency of a specific apolipoprotein (apoEIII) in the very-low-density lipoproteins. *FEBS Letters* **56:** 352–5.

Vagelos R, Galambos L. (2004) *Medicine, Science and Merck.* Cambridge; New York, NY: Cambridge University Press.

Vasile E, Simionescu M, Simionescu N. (1983) Visualization of the binding, endocytosis, and transcytosis of low-density lipoprotein in the arterial endothelium in situ. *Journal of Cell Biology* **96:** 1677–89.

Venn B J, Mann J I. (2004) Cereal grains, legumes and diabetes. *European Journal of Clinical Nutrition* **58:** 1443–61.

Walker J F, Tobert J A. (1987) The clinical efficacy and safety of lovastatin and MK-733: an overview. *European Heart Journal* **8** Suppl E: 93–6.

Walton K W, Scott P J. (1964) Estimation of the low-density (beta) lipoproteins of serum in health and disease using large molecular weight dextran sulphate. *Journal of Clinical Pathology* **17:** 627–43.

Watts G F, Lewis B, Brunt J N, Lewis E S, Coltart D J, Smith L D, Mann J I, Swan A V. (1992) Effects on coronary artery disease of lipid-lowering diet, or diet plus cholestyramine, in the St Thomas' Atherosclerosis Regression Study (STARS). *Lancet* **339:** 563–9.

Weisgraber K H, Innerarity T L, Mahley R W. (1978) Role of lysine residues of plasma lipoproteins in high affinity binding to cell surface receptors on human fibroblasts. *Journal of Biological Chemistry* **253:** 9053–62.

West of Scotland Coronary Prevention Study Group (WOSCOPS). (1995) Screening experience and baseline characteristics in the West of Scotland Coronary Prevention Study. The West of Scotland Coronary Prevention Study. *American Journal of Cardiology* **76:** 485–91.

West of Scotland Coronary Prevention Study Group (WOSCOPS). (1997) Baseline risk factors and their association with outcome in the West of Scotland Coronary Prevention Study. *American Journal of Cardiology* **79:** 756–62.

Westlund K, Nicolaysen R. (1966) Serum cholesterol and risk of mortality and morbidity. A 3-year follow-up of 6886 men. *Scandinavian Journal of Clinical and Laboratory Investigation, Supplementum* **87:** 1–19.

White P D. (1947) *Heart Disease.* 3rd edn. New York, NY: Macmillan.

Wilkes H C, Meade T W, Barzegar S, Foley A J, Hughes L O, Bauer K A, Rosenberg R D, Miller G J. (1992) Gemfibrozil reduces plasma prothrombin fragment F1 + 2 concentration, a marker of coagulability, in patients with coronary heart disease. *Thrombosis and Haemostasis* **67:** 503–6.

Wood P H. (1950) *Diseases of the Heart and Circulation. The Practitioner* series. London: Eyre and Spottiswoode.

Woolf N, Pilkington T R. (1965) The immunohistochemical demonstration of lipoproteins in vessel walls. *Journal of Pathology and Bacteriology* **90:** 459–63.

Wright H P. (1941) Adhesiveness of blood platelets in normal subjects with varying concentration of anticoagulants. *Journal of Pathology and Bacteriology* **53:** 255–62.

Wright L D, Cresson E L, Skeggs H R, MacRae G D E, Hoffman C H, Wolf D E, Folkers K. (1956) Isolation of a new acetate-replacing factor. *Journal of the American Chemical Society* **78:** 5273–5.

Writing Group for the Women's Health Initiative Investigators. (2002) Risks and benefits of estrogen plus progestin in healthy postmenopausal women: Principal results from the Women's Health Initiative Randomized Controlled Trial. *Journal of the American Medical Association* **288:** 321–33.

Yudkin J. (1958) *This Slimming Business*. London: MacGibbon and Kee.

Yudkin J. (1964) Dietary fat and dietary sugar in relation to ischaemic heart disease and diabetes. *Lancet* **41:** 4–5.

Yudkin J. (1972) *Pure, White and Deadly: The problem of sugar*. London: Davis-Poynter.

Yudkin J. (1974) Why suspicion falls on sugar as a major cause of heart disease. *The Times* (11 July): 16.

Yudkin J. (1985) *The Penguin Encyclopedia of Nutrition*. Harmondsworth: Viking.

Yudkin J S. (1993) Circulating proinsulin-like molecules. *Journal of Diabetes and its Complications* **7:** 113–23.

Yudkin J S. (2000) Relationship of serum C3 complement with insulin resistance and coronary heart disease – cause, consequence or common antecedent? *European Heart Journal* **21:** 1036–9.

Yudkin J S, May M, Elwood P, Yarnell J W, Greenwood R, Davey Smith G (Caerphilly Study). (2002) Concentrations of proinsulin like molecules predict coronary heart disease risk independently of insulin: prospective data from the Caerphilly Study. *Diabetologia* **45:** 327–36.

Zannis V I, Just P W, Breslow J L. (1981) Human apolipoprotein E isoprotein subclasses are genetically determined. *American Journal of Human Genetics* **33:** 11–24.

Biographical notes*

Professor David Barker
CBE MD PhD FRCP FRS (b. 1938) has been Professor of Clinical Epidemiology at the University of Southampton since 1972, and Professor in the Department of Medicine of the Oregon Health in Science University, USA, since 2003. From 1982–2003 he was Director of the MRC Environmental Epidemiology Unit at the University of Southampton.

Professor John Betteridge
MD PhD FRCP (b. 1948) is Professor of Endocrinology and Metabolism at the Royal Free and University College School of Medicine, London. He was appointed honorary physician to University College Hospital in 1981. He is a past chairman of the British Hyperlipidaemia Association (now HEART UK) and a past president of the Royal Society of Medicine's section on lipids in clinical medicine. He was R D Lawrence Fellow of the British Diabetic Association (now Diabetes UK).

Sir Christopher Booth
Kt FRCP (b. 1924) trained as a gastroenterologist and was Professor of Medicine at the Royal Postgraduate Medical School, Hammersmith Hospital, London, from 1966 to 1977 and Director of the Medical Research Council's Clinical Research Centre, Northwick Park Hospital, Harrow, from 1978 to 1988. He was the first Convenor of the Wellcome Trust's History of Twentieth Century Medicine Group, from 1990 to 1996, and Harveian Librarian at the Royal College of Physicians from 1989 to 1997.

Professor Gustav Born
FRCP HonFRCS FRS (b. 1921) was Vandervell Professor of Pharmacology at the Royal College of Surgeons from 1960 to 1973; Sheild Professor of Pharmacology at the University of Cambridge, and Fellow of Gonville and Caius College, Cambridge, from 1973 to 1978 and Professor of Pharmacology at King's College, London, from 1978 to 1986, later Emeritus. He is currently Research Professor at the William Harvey Research Institute, Bart's and the

* Contributors are asked to supply details; other entries are compiled from conventional biographical sources.

Royal London School of Medicine and Dentistry, University of London. He was the Founding President of the British Society of Haemostasis and Thrombosis from 1979 to 1981. One of the handmade aggregometers is in the Düsseldorf Academy of Science Museum. For further details of his work with the optical aggregometer, see Reynolds and Tansey (eds) (2005).

Professor George Boyd
PhD FRSE (1924–83) educated at Heriot-Watt and Edinburgh University, he obtained his PhD in 1951 and became a lecturer in biochemistry with Professor Guy Marrian FRS. He worked on cholesterol metabolism with Michael Oliver until 1960, when he became a senior lecturer in biochemistry, receiving a personal chair in 1970 and in 1976 became Chairman of the University of Edinburgh Department of Biochemistry until his death in 1983. From 1969, he was Director of the MRC Group on Sterol Metabolism, a member of the MRC Physiological Systems Board, 1980–83, and Vice-President of the Royal Society of Edinburgh from 1980–83.

Professor Sydney Brenner
CH FRCP Hon FRCPath FRS (b. 1927) shared the 2002 Nobel Prize in Physiology or Medicine equally with H Robert Horvitz and John E Sulston 'for their discoveries concerning genetic regulation of organ development and programmed cell death'. He qualified at the University of Witwatersrand and Oxford, was a member of the scientific staff of the Medical Research Council from 1957 to 1992, and a Fellow of King's College, Cambridge, since 1959. He directed the MRC Laboratory of Molecular Biology, Cambridge from 1979 to 1986 and the MRC Molecular Genetics Unit, Cambridge, 1986 to 1992, when he moved to the Scripps Research Institute in La Jolla, California, in 1992, becoming President and Director of Research at the Molecular Sciences Institute, Berkeley, from 1996 to 2001. He has been Distinguished Research Professor at the Salk Institute, La Jolla, since 2001. In 2000 he was awarded the Albert Lasker Award for Special Achievement. See Brenner (2001).

Professor Brian Bronte-Stewart
MD MRCP (1923–65) qualified in medicine in 1944 at the University of Cape Town, South Africa, and trained at Groote Schuur Hospital, Cape Town. He started research into the role of cholesterol in the causation of atheroma while at St Mary's Hospital, London

under Sir George Pickering and later with Ancel Keys on dietary influences on cholesterol. In 1961, Sir Harold Himsworth persuaded him to become Director of the newly established Medical Research Council Atheroma Research Unit in the Western Infirmary, Glasgow, for four years until his death from cancer at the age of 42 in 1965.

Professor Michael Brown MD (b. 1941) graduated in chemistry from the University of Pennsylvania and in 1966 met Joseph L Goldstein, a fellow intern in Internal Medicine at the Massachusetts General Hospital in Boston. He was at the National Institutes of Health, from 1968, moving to the division of gastroenterology in the Department of Internal Medicine, University of Texas Southwestern Medical School, Dallas, in 1971. There he succeeded in solubilizing and partially purifying an enzyme that catalyses the rate-controlling enzyme in cholesterol biosynthesis. He and Goldstein developed the hypothesis that abnormalities in the regulation of this enzyme were the cause of familial hypercholesterolaemia, and began collaborating in 1972 in Dallas, although their separate laboratories did not join until 1974. Brown was appointed Professor of Internal Medicine in 1976 and a year later as Paul Thomas Professor of Medicine and Genetics and Director of the Center for Genetic Disease, and he became Regental Professor of the University of Texas in 1985. Brown and Goldstein shared the Nobel Prize for Physiology or Medicine in 1985, as well as numerous other awards. See http://nobelprize.org/medicine/laureates/1985/brown-bio.html (visited 2 November 2005). See Figure 2.

Professor Richard Bruckdorfer PhD DSc (b. 1942) was educated at the University of Liverpool and held postdoctoral positions at the Universities of Utrecht and Munich, and then at Queen Elizabeth College, London. He was appointed lecturer in biochemistry at the Royal Free Hospital School of Medicine, and Professor of Biochemistry in 1995, and remains in that post at UCL. His original work was on the role of cholesterol in cell membranes, but increasingly became interested in oxidation of lipids and lipoproteins related to atherosclerosis and, in particular, its effects on nitric oxide biology.

Professor George Davey Smith MSc MD DSc FFPHM FRCP (b. 1959) has been Professor of Clinical Epidemiology in the Department of Social Medicine at the University of Bristol since 1994.

Professor Michael Davies
MD FRCPath (1937–2003) qualified at Middlesex Hospital Medical School, London, was appointed registrar in pathology in 1963 at St George's Hospital and Medical School, London, later senior lecturer in pathology, reader in cardiac pathology, was appointed to a personal chair in cardiac pathology in 1977 and was the first British Heart Foundation Professor of Cardiovascular Pathology from 1981 until his retirement in 2001. He was editor of *Heart* (formerly the *British Heart Journal*), 1991–99, and a founder member of the European School for Cardiovascular Pathology (now the Association for European Cardiovascular Pathologists) from 1994.

Professor Paul Durrington
MD FRCP FRCPath FMedSci (b. 1947) is a physician, who has been Professor of Medicine at the University of Manchester since 1995. His interest in lipoprotein metabolism began in 1974 with his MD studies on apolipoprotein B in Bristol. In 1979–80 he was a Travelling Fellow of the British Heart Foundation at the University of California, San Diego, investigating insulin and hepatic lipoprotein secretion. He was elected to the Fellowship of the Academy of Medical Sciences in 2001 for his work on dyslipidaemia and HDL metabolism.

Lord Howard Florey
Bt OM FRS (1898–1968), Australian-born experimental pathologist and the main creator of penicillin therapy, studied blood flow in brain capillaries under Sir Charles Sherrington at Oxford, at the pathology department in Cambridge, and in the US. He was appointed Huddersfield lecturer in pathology, Cambridge, in 1927; Joseph Hunter Professor of Pathology, Sheffield, in 1932; and succeeded Georges Dreyer as Professor of Pathology, Oxford, from 1935 to 1962, later Emeritus. He carried out research with (Sir) Ernst Chain on penicillin, and its effectiveness was proved on patients at the Radcliffe Infirmary, Oxford, 1941–42, and on war wounds in North Africa with (Sir) Hugh Cairns in 1943. He shared the Nobel Prize for Physiology or Medicine in 1945 for the discovery and development of penicillin with Sir Alexander Fleming Kt FRCP FRS (1881–1955), and Sir Ernst Chain Kt FRS (1906–1979). See Florey (ed.) (1970).

Dr John E French
DPhil, collaborated with Lord Florey and was University Demonstrator in Pathology at Sir William Dunn School of Pathology, University of Oxford.

Dr W F M (Bill) Fulton
BSc MD FRCP (b. 1919), responsible for unique and pioneering studies on coronary arteries using stereoarteriography, serially-mounted 2mm transverse sections, selective histopathology and their relation to clinical events. He was Research Assistant in Cardiology at the University of Edinburgh from 1952–53, Consultant Physician, Stobhill General Hospital, Glasgow, and Reader, Department of Materia Medica, University of Glasgow from 1958 to 1984. Other appointments include Senior Fellow in Cardiology, the Johns Hopkins Hospital, Baltimore, Maryland, 1963–64, and Foundation Professor of Medicine, University of Nairobi, Kenya, 1967–72. See Figure 4.

Professor David Galton
FRCP (b. 1937) was Professor and head of the Department of Human Metabolism and Molecular Genetics at St Bartholomew's Hospital, London, from 1971 to 2002, later Emeritus. He has been Professor Emeritus at the Wolfson Institute of Preventive Medicine, London, since 2003. See Galton (2003).

Professor Joseph Goldstein
MD (b. 1940) trained at Washington and Lee University in Lexington, Virginia, and Southwestern Medical School of the University of Texas Health Science Center, Dallas. Before returning to Dallas he worked with Arno Motulsky at the University of Washington in Seattle, where he and his colleagues discovered that 20 per cent of all heart attack survivors have one of three single-gene determined types of hereditary hyperlipidaemia, including heterozygous FH. In 1972 he persuaded Brown to join him in Dallas when he was appointed Assistant Professor and head of the medical schools' first Division of Medical Genetics, later Associate Professor of Internal Medicine in 1974, Professor in 1976, and Chairman of the Department of Molecular Genetics at the University of Texas Health Science Center at Dallas and Paul J Thomas Professor of Medicine and Genetics a year later. Brown and Goldstein shared the Nobel Prize for Physiology or Medicine in 1985. See http://nobelprize.org/medicine/laureates/1985/goldstein-bio.html (visited 2 November 2005). See Figure 2.

Professor Antonio (Tony) Gotto, Jr
MD DPhil, researcher in the field of lipid chemistry and the role of lipoproteins in cholesterol metabolism, has been Dean and Provost for Medical Affairs at Cornell University and Weill Medical College, New York, NY, since 1997. He was a Rhodes Scholar at Oxford University, trained in internal medicine at Massachusetts General Hospital, Boston, Massachusetts. He served in the US Public Health Service at the National Institutes of Health, 1967–69, and then as a Research Associate of the National Heart, Lung and Blood Institute. From 1971 to 1996, he was Professor of Medicine and Biochemistry at Baylor College of Medicine in Houston, Texas, and Chairman of Internal Medicine there from 1977 to 1996. See Figure 2.

Sir Harold Himsworth
KCB FRCP FRS (1905–93), a distinguished clinical scientist, was appointed Professor of Medicine and Director of the Medical Unit at University College Hospital (UCH), London, in 1939, a post he held until appointed Secretary of the Medical Research Council (MRC) from 1949 to 1968. Although MRC Secretary, he was not a member of the Medical Research Council until 1957. His major project, the Clinical Research Centre at Northwick Park, Harrow, was inspired by Sir Thomas Lewis [Gray and Booth (1994): 240.].

Dr Arthur Hollman
MD FRCP FLS (b. 1923) was Consultant Cardiologist at University College Hospital, London, from 1962 until his retirement in 1988. He has been Honorary Consultant Cardiologist at the Conquest Hospital, Hastings, East Sussex, since 2001, and the Archivist to the British Cardiac Society since 1992.

Professor Steve Humphries
PhD FRCPath MRCP (b. 1950) was educated at the Universities of Sussex and Glasgow, and held postdoctoral positions in Glasgow, Utah and at St Mary's Hospital Medical School, London, before moving in 1985 to the British Heart Foundation-funded research team at the Charing Cross Sunley Research Centre as Senior Lecturer, later Reader and Professor in the University of London. He has been Professor of Cardiovascular Genetics at the Royal Free and University College Hospital Medical School, London, since 1991. He was one of the first to recognize that pathophysiological insights could be gained through identifying functional candidate gene variants,

and determining their effect in healthy subjects, focusing on gene-environment interactions, the key to understanding the multifactorial nature of heart disease.

Professor Ancel Keys
PhD PhD (1904–2004), an American scientist who studied the influence of different kinds of dietary fat on health, also called 'Mr Cholesterol', was educated at the University of California, Berkeley, in economics and political science and biology, with PhDs in oceanography and biology (1930) and physiology (1938) from the University of Cambridge, UK. He was appointed Professor at the University of Minnesota in 1936, where he established the Laboratory of Physiological Hygiene, and was its Director from 1939 until his retirement in 1972. He designed the K-ration, investigated the physiological effects of starvation on humans [Keys *et al.* (1950)], was on the cover of *Time* magazine (31 January 1961), undertook the first prospective study of cardiovascular disease, among Minnesota businessmen [Keys *et al.* (1963)], and later the Seven Countries study [Keys (1980)]. For a discussion of his work, see www.asph.org/movies/keys.pdf (visited 16 February 2006).

Sir Thomas Lewis
CBE FRCP FRS (1881–1945), cardiologist and clinical scientist, directed the first of the MRC's research units, the Clinical Research Department, established at University College Hospital Medical School, London, from 1919 until his retirement in 1945. He was awarded the first Beit Fellowships in 1910. See Lewis (1932, 1946); for further details of his appointment to UCL, see Himsworth (1982); and Drury and Grant (1945–48). A collection of his papers, CMAC/PP/LEW, is held in Archives and Manuscripts, Wellcome Library, London.

Dame June Lloyd
DBE MD FRCP FRCPE FRCGP DPH (b. 1928) trained at the Universities of Bristol and Durham, with posts in medicine and paediatrics at Bristol, Oxford, Newcastle and Birmingham from 1951–65. She was appointed senior lecturer at the Institute of Child Health, London, in 1969, followed by reader in 1969 and professor in 1974. She was Professor at St George's Medical School, London, from 1975–85 and Nuffield Professor of Child Health in the University of London from 1985 until her retirement in 1992. She was scientific adviser to the Association of Medical Research Charities; Chairman of the Gene

Therapy Advisory Committee, and past paediatric vice-president of the Royal College of Physicians of London.

Professor Gordon Lowe
MD FRCP (b. 1949) trained in general medicine, haemostasis and thrombosis in Nottingham and Glasgow. He was appointed Senior Lecturer in Medicine at the University of Glasgow and Honorary Consultant Physician at the Glasgow Royal Infirmary in 1985 and has been Professor of Vascular Medicine there since 1993.

Professor Jim Mann
PhD DM FFPHM FRACP (b. 1944) has been Professor of Human Nutrition and Medicine, University of Otago, Dunedin, New Zealand, since 1988. A physician, he trained in Cape Town, South Africa and Oxford, and worked in Oxford as University Lecturer in Social and Community Medicine, Honorary Consultant Physician and Fellow of Wolfson College from 1972 to 1988.

Professor Vincent Marks
MA DM FRCP FRCPath (b. 1930) trained at St Thomas' Hospital Medical School, was Senior Lecturer in Chemical Pathology at the Institute of Neurology, London, from 1958 to 1962. He was Consultant Chemical Pathologist at the Epsom Group of Hospitals from 1962 to 1970. He was appointed Professor of Clinical Biochemistry at the University of Surrey from 1970 until his retirement in 1995, later Emeritus.

Professor Sir Michael Marmot
Kt PhD MPH FRCP MPH FMedSci (b. 1945), an international authority on social inequalities in health, has been Professor of Epidemiology and Public Health at the Royal Free and University College Medical School, London, since 1985 and Director of the International Centre for Health and Society, UCL, since 1994. He was the co-architect of the Whitehall Civil Servants Studies and Chairman of the third Report of the DHSS COMA Panel on Diet in relation to Cardiovascular Disease.

Dr Archer (John Porter) Martin
FRS (1910–2002) was educated at Cambridge University and the Physical Chemistry Laboratory, moving to the Dunn Nutritional Laboratory, and in 1938 to the Wool Industries Research Association at Leeds, and later Head of the Biochemistry Division of the Research Department of Boots Pure Drug Company at Nottingham, 1946–48. He joined the staff of the Medical Research Council in 1948, first at the Lister Institute and in 1950 at the National Institute for

Medical Research. He headed the Division of Physical Chemistry in 1952 and was Chemical Consultant from 1956 to 1959, when he became Director of Abbotsbury Laboratories Ltd. At the Wool Industries Research Association he worked on the felting of wool and on amino-acid analysis. It was here that he developed his method of partition chromatography; later, with A T James, he developed the method of gas–liquid chromatography. See note 224.

Professor Sir John McMichael
FRS (1904–93) was Professor and Director of the Department of Medicine at the Postgraduate Medical School at Hammersmith between 1946 and 1966, then directed the British Postgraduate Medical Federation from 1966 to 1971. His research interests were predominantly in the field of cardiology and he was the first in Britain to apply the technique of cardiac catheterization. See Dollery (1995).

Dr Clarence Merskey
FRCP (1914–82) worked with Rosemary Biggs and Gwyn Macfarlane from 1949 to 1951 at the Radcliffe Infirmary, Oxford, where he developed his coagulation expertise and made valuable contributions to the study of haemophilia. In New York he collaborated closely with Alan Johnson devising tests for measuring fibrin degradation products. For further aspects of his work, see Tansey and Christie (eds) (1999): 5, 9–10, 44–45.

Dr Norman Miller
MB PhD FRCP along with George Miller, he published the HDL hypothesis in 1975. He later participated in the Tromso Heart Study in Norway, and spent two years at the Baker Heart Research Institute, Melbourne, Australia. He was appointed Reader in Metabolic Disease at St Thomas' Hospital Medical School, London, from 1978 to 1987; Professor of Medicine and Head of Endocrinology and Metabolism at Bowman Gray School of Medicine at Wake Forest University, Winston-Salem, North Carolina, for four years; and from 1992 to 2002 was British Heart Foundation Professor of Cardiovascular Biochemistry at St Bartholomew's Hospital Medical School, London. He is Adjunct Professor of Internal Medicine and Visiting Professor in Cardiovascular Genetics, University of Utah School of Medicine, Salt Lake City, Utah.

Dr Paul Miller
MSc DPhil FRCP (b. 1940) is Consultant Gastroenterologist to the South Manchester University

Hospitals, where he started the Lipid Clinic in 1975. As an MRC Travelling Fellow he spent a period in lipoprotein research at Baylor College of Medicine, Houston, Texas, and was a founder member of the Committee of the British Hyperlipidaemia Society (now HEART UK). He was until recently Chairman of the Council of the Medical Protection Society.

Professor J R A (Tony) Mitchell (1928–91) was Foundation Professor of Medicine at the University of Nottingham, from 1968 to 1990. See H(ampton) J R (1991); Mitchell (1987).

Professor Jerry Morris CBE DSc DPH Hon MD FRCP (b. 1910) was Director of the MRC Social Medicine Research Unit from 1948 to 1975, initially as a member of staff of the Medical Research Council from 1948 to 1966 and then also as Professor of Public Health, University of London, at the London Hospital and the London School of Hygiene and Tropical Medicine from 1966 to 1978, later Emeritus. See a video recording of Jerry Morris in interview with Max Blythe, [Oxford Brookes University, 1986] held as 1856V, in the Moving Image and Sound Collection of the Wellcome Library, London. See also Davey Smith (2004).

Dr Nicolas (Nick) Myant DM FRCP (b. 1917) qualified at Oxford and University College Hospital, London, and was Sir Thomas Lewis's House Physician in 1943. He was Director of the MRC Lipid Metabolism Unit at the Hammersmith Hospital, London, from 1969 to 1983. The British Hyperlipidaemia Association has supported an annual Myant Lecture since 1989 in recognition of his influential role in lipid research in Britain during the 1960s and 1970s at the Hammersmith Hospital, supported by the Medical Research Council. See, for example, Myant (1990a and b, 1993). See also Introduction and Figure 2.

Professor Michael Oliver CBE MD MDhc (Karolinska and Bologna) FRCP FRSE (b. 1925) was the Duke of Edinburgh Professor of Cardiology at the University of Edinburgh from 1976 to 1989, later Emeritus. He was President of the British Cardiac Society from 1980 to 1984; of the Royal College of Physicians of Edinburgh from 1986 to 1988; and Director of the Wynn Institute for Metabolic Research from 1990 to 1994. He served on the COMA and MAFF Committees; and was the UK representative on the Cardiovascular Division of WHO, 1955–2000.

Professor Chris Packard
PhD DSc FRCPath FRCP(Gla) FRSE (b. 1953) has been honorary professor in the Faculty of Medicine at University of Glasgow since 1995 and also works part of the time as a clinical scientist investigating the causes and treatment of heart disease, as well as the R&D Director for the North Glasgow University Hospitals Division of the Greater Glasgow Health Board. He was study director of the West of Scotland Coronary Prevention Study [Shepherd *et al.* (1995)] and the Prospective Study of Pravastatin in the Elderly at Risk [Shepherd *et al.* (1999)], trials that established statins as primary prevention and in the elderly. He is also founding chairman of Nexxus, the West of Scotland Bioscience Network, which promotes community building and knowledge exchange between the life sciences industry, academia and the NHS.

Professor Stuart Pocock
is Professor of Medical Statistics at the London School of Hygiene and Tropical Medicine, London, and Director of the Clinical Trials Research Group.

Professor Kalevi Pyörälä
FRCP (b. 1930) was Associate Professor of Medicine at the University of Helsinki from 1969 to 1975, Research Professor at the Academy of Finland from 1973 to 1975 and Professor of Medicine at the University of Kuopio from 1975 to 1993, later Emeritus.

Professor Gerald Reaven
MD, Emeritus Professor of Medicine at Stanford University, first described Syndrome X at the 1988 Banting Lecture of the annual meeting of the American Diabetes Association. He served as Director of the Division of Endocrinology and Metabolism, the Division of Gerontology, and the combined Divisions of Endocrinology–Metabolism–Gerontology at Stanford's School of Medicine, California. See Reaven (1988).

Professor Geoffrey Rose
CBE DM FRCP FRCGP FFPHM (1926–93) was Professor of Epidemiology at St Mary's Hospital Medical School from 1970 to 1977; at the London School of Hygiene and Tropical Medicine from 1977 until his retirement in 1991, later Emeritus; and Honorary Consultant Physician, St Mary's Hospital, 1964–91. He had been Chairman of the WHO Expert Committees on Heart Disease Prevention, 1982 and 1984; and of the Council on Epidemiology and Prevention, International Society and Federation of Cardiology, 1982–86. See Barker and Rose (1976, 1979, 1984, 1990).

Professor William Rutter
(b. 1928), biochemist and biotechnologist, joined the Department of Biochemistry and Biophysics, University of California, San Francisco (UCSF) as Professor and chairman of the department from 1968 to 1982 and Director of the Hormone Research Institute, UCSF from 1983 to 1994. For further details of his work, see a 1992 interview, freely available at http://content.cdlib.org/xtf/view?docId=kt7q2nb2hm&doc.view=entire_text&brand=oac (visited 27 February 2006).

Professor Tom Sanders
DSc (b. 1949), educated at the University of London, was appointed Professor of Nutrition and Dietetics at King's College London in 1994 and is now Head of the Research Division of Nutritional Sciences there.

Professor James Scott
FRCP FIBiol FMedSci FRS (b. 1946), trained at the London Hospital and in Birmingham, was appointed to the Academic Department of Medicine at the Royal Free Hospital, London, in 1975; an MRC Research Fellow and Honorary Senior Registrar at the Royal Postgraduate Medical School, Hammersmith Hospital, London, 1975–80; European Molecular Biology Fellow at the Department of Biochemistry, University of California, San Francisco, 1980–83 and MRC Clinical Scientist and Honorary Consultant Physician at the MRC Clinical Research Centre, Northwick Park Hospital, from 1983 to 1991. He has been Honorary Consultant Physician at the Hammersmith Hospital since 1992; Professor and Chairman of Medicine at the Royal Postgraduate Medical School, Hammersmith Hospital, from 1992 to 1998; and Director of the Genetics and Genomics Institute, Imperial College, and Professor of Cardiovascular Medicine National Heart and Lung Institute, Medicine, London, since 1998.

Sir Ernest Henry Shackleton
Kt (1874–1922), explorer, went to the South Pole with Scott's National Antarctic Expedition on the Discovery expedition in 1901. He commanded the Nimrod Expedition (1907–9), and the 1914–16 voyage on *HMS Endurance.* He died while attempting to circumnavigate the Antarctic continent on South Georgia Island where his wife insisted he be buried.

Professor A G (Gerry) Shaper
FRCP FRCPath (b. 1927) qualified in Cape Town, joining the Department of Medicine at Makerere University Medical School, Kampala, Uganda, in

1957, moving to the MRC Social Medicine Unit at the London School of Hygiene and Tropical Medicine in 1970 and in 1975 to the Department of Epidemiology and Public Health as Professor of Clinical Epidemiology at the Royal Free Hospital School of Medicine, London, until his retirement in 1992, later Emeritus.

Dr Hugh Sinclair
DM DSc FRCP (1910–90), an eccentric nutritionist, was educated at Winchester College and Magdalen College, Oxford. He pioneered work on vitamins and essential fatty acids and was Vice-President of Magdalen College. He established the Chair of Human Nutrition at the University of Reading. See Ewin (2001).

Dr Joan Slack
DM DCH FRCP (b. 1925) educated at St Hilda's College, Oxford, followed by an NIH Foreign Fellowship in biochemical genetics at the Children's Memorial Hospital, Chicago, Illinois, 1959–60. She was a member of the MRC Clinical Genetics Research Unit at the Institute of Child Health, London, from 1960–72 and Consultant in Clinical Genetics at St Mark's and the Royal Free Hospitals, London, 1975–90. Her early studies included lipoprotein lipase activity in children with cystic fibrosis and CHD in familial hypercholesterolaemia. See Figure 2.

Dr Elspeth Bruce Smith
PhD DSc FRS(E) (b. 1923)[née Dunkerley], was educated at Cambridge, London and Aberdeen. She worked in the Ministry of Aircraft Production during the war, was a research assistant at Cambridge and St Bartholomew's Hospital, London, until appointed Senior Lecturer at the Middlesex Hospital, London, in 1955, moving to the University of Aberdeen in 1968 as Lecturer and later Reader.

Professor Anne Soutar
PhD (b. 1945) educated as a biochemist and enzymologist, she has been a research programme leader in the Medical Research Council's Clinical Sciences Centre, Imperial College at the Hammersmith Hospital, London, since 1993. Her career in lipoprotein research started in the early 1970s with a postdoctoral fellowship with Tony Gotto, at Baylor College of Medicine, Houston, Texas.

Professor Siegfried Thannhauser
MD PhD (1885–1962) trained in medicine and biochemistry in Munich and was appointed assistant physician at the Hospital of the Ludwig-Maximilans-University in 1912. After

military service, he directed the Departments of Medicine at Heidelberg, Dusseldorf and Freiburg from 1924 to 1934, before being dismissed by the Nazi government. He practised privately in Freiburg until the Rockefeller Foundation arranged an offer of the post of Associate Clinical Professor, later Clinical Professor, at Tufts University, Boston, and Senior Physician at the New England Medical Centre, Boston, Massachusetts, from 1937 until his death in 1962. He was also Director of the Thannhauser Research Laboratory at the Boston Dispensary.

Professor Gilbert Thompson
MD FRCP (b. 1932) qualified at St Thomas' Hospital Medical School, London, in 1956. Following military service he joined the Royal Postgraduate Medical School, Hammersmith Hospital, London, in 1963, where he remained until1998, with periods of research spent at the Massachusetts General Hospital, Boston, Massachusetts; the Methodist Hospital, Houston, Texas; and the Royal Victoria Hospital, Montreal, Quebec, Canada, where he was the recipient of the Lucien Award in 1982. He led the MRC Lipoprotein team at the Hammersmith Hospital, London and was Honorary Consultant Physician in charge of the lipid clinic from 1993–98; was a past Chairman of both the British Hyperlipidaemia Association and the British Atherosclerosis Society, and has been Emeritus Professor in Clinical Lipidology at Imperial College, London, since 1998. See Figure 2.

Dr Jonathan Tobert
MB BChir PhD (b. 1945) was a member of Merck Research Laboratories in Rahway, New Jersey, from 1976 until his retirement in 2004 as Executive Director, Department of Clinical Endocrinology and Metabolism. He is an honorary consultant to the Clinical Trials Service Unit, Nuffield Department of Medicine, University of Oxford.

Professor Hugh Tunstall-Pedoe
MD FRCP FRCPE FFPH FESC (b. 1939) trained in cardiology and general medicine before taking up cardiovascular epidemiology in 1969, working with Professor Jerry Morris in the MRC Social Medicine Unit and then with Professor Geoffrey Rose at St Mary's Hospital Medical School, London, in 1974. He was Professor and Director of the Cardiovascular Epidemiology Unit at the University of Dundee from 1981 to 2005, later Emeritus. See Tunstall-Pedoe (ed.) (2003).

Professor Hubert Maitland Turnbull
FRCP FRS (1875–1955) qualified and trained at the London Hospital; was a Radcliffe Travelling Fellow in Copenhagen and Dresden, where his work as a voluntary assistant with Professor Georg Schmorl in Dresden determined his interest in pathology. He directed the Institute of Pathology, London Hospital, from 1906 to 1946, becoming Reader in Morbid Anatomy in the University of London in 1915 and Professor in 1919, later Emeritus. His meticulous care in the observation and recording of details at post mortem gave pathology a scientific basis. Much of his work appeared under his students' names and his reputation ensured that the Institute of Pathology had a full quota of voluntary assistants. Anonymous (1968); Turnbull (1920).

Professor Paul Dudley White
MD FRCP (1886–1973), American cardiac physician, qualified at Harvard and trained at the Massachusetts General Hospital, Boston, and University College Hospital Medical School, London. He taught at Harvard Medical School from 1914–20; was Professor of Medicine and physician in charge of the cardiac clinics and laboratory, from 1919 to 1949. A founder of the American Heart Association, he served as President, 1940–42; and received the Albert Lasker award in 1953. See White (1947, 1950).

Dr Paul Hamilton Wood
OBE MD FRCP (1907–62) trained at Melbourne University, did house jobs at Christchurch Hospital, New Zealand; Brompton Hospital, London; the National Heart Hospital, London, and the British Postgraduate Medical School, London, where he was First Assistant from 1935–40 and senior lecturer, 1946–48, after war service. He was Dean of the Institute of Cardiology, 1947–50, Cardiologist at the Rheumatic Fever Unit, Canadian Red Cross Memorial Hospital, Taplow, 1947–53, and Director of the Institute of Cardiology, London; Physician, National Heart Hospital, London; Physician, Cardiac Department, Brompton Hospital, London, from 1953–62. See Wood (1950).

Professor Neville Woolf
FRCPath (b. 1930), born and educated in Cape Town, South Africa, he came to Britain in 1959, was appointed Reader in Experimental Pathology at St George's Hospital Medical School, London, before moving to the Middlesex Hospital Medical School as Bland-Sutton Professor of

Histopathology in 1975. Following the merger of the Middlesex and University College Hospital Medical Schools, London, in 1982, he became head of the joint department of histopathology until 1987. He retired from his chair in 1995, and was Vice-Dean and Faculty Tutor in the Faculty of Clinical Sciences at UCL until 2004, at which time he became Emeritus.

Professor John Yudkin
(1910–92), Professor of Nutrition at Queen Elizabeth College, London, from 1954 until his retirement in 1971, later Emeritus, trained at Cambridge and the London Hospital. He worked at the Biochemical Laboratory, Cambridge, 1931–36; the Nutritional Laboratory, Cambridge, 1938–43; and was Professor of Physiology, Queen Elizabeth College, London, 1945–54. In 1953 Yudkin was responsible for the first comprehensive university courses leading to Bachelor's and Master's degrees in nutrition. He was Chairman of the Food Group, Society of Chemical Industry. See, for example, Yudkin (1958, 1972, 1985).

Professor John S Yudkin
MD FRCP (b. 1943) has been Professor of Medicine at UCL since 1992 and Director of the International Health and Medical Education Centre in the Diabetes and Cardiovascular Disease Academic Unit at the Royal Free and University College Medical School since 2000. He is interested in novel risk factors for cardiovascular disease, including insulin resistance and low-grade inflammation.

Glossary*

aldehyde
An organic compound with a double bond between a carbon atom and an oxygen stem, containing the aldehydric group, with at least one hydrogen attached to it. Lipoperoxidation-derived aldehydes, for example malondialdehyde (MDA), can damage proteins.

antioxidants
Substances that reduce oxidative damage caused by free radicals.

apolipoprotein (A, B, C, E, etc.)
A protein found integrally associated with plasma lipoproteins.

arteriosclerosis
A term used in the past to describe generalized hardening of the arteries.

atherosclerosis
The term commonly used to describe the partially occlusive lesions that occur in the inner lining of arteries when there is cholesterol deposit and thrombosis.

atorvastatin
(*Lipitor*®, Parke, Davis and Co.) A statin. Licensed in the UK in 1996 as a prescription-only medicine.

autosomal recessive disorder
Caused by an error or mutation in a single unit of genetic information, a recessive disorder will be expressed in a person only if both copies of the gene are mutated.

carrier
An unaffected person who harbours a disease gene.

chlorophenoxyisobutyrate (CPIB)
The active principle of clofibrate.

cholesterol nomenclature, types I–V
Described by Fredrickson in 1966 and now rarely used (Fredrickson *et al.* (1966): 429–88).

cholesterol readings
Normal values [in early 2006] for cholesterol, depending upon age and gender, are: 140–220mg/dl (US, which measures the mass in milligrammes); 3.6–5.7mmol/l (SI [Système Internationale] units measures concentrations in terms of the number of particles or moles present). To convert one to the other, multiply mg/dl by 0.0259 to obtain mmol/l units. [Lewis *et al.* (1992): Table B-1, 1818.] For population readings, see Section 9.3.2, *Health Survey of England*

*We are grateful to Professors Michael Oliver and Chris Packard for assistance in compiling this glossary.

2003, following links at www.dh.gov.uk/assetRoot/04/09/89/11/04098911.pdf (visited 9 March 2006).

cholestyramine
A resin taken by mouth which is not itself absorbed but which acts to interfere with the reabsorption of bile acids in the gut. For example, *Questran*® (Bristol-Myers Squibb).

clofibrate (*Atromid-S* ®, ICI)
A broad-spectrum, lipid-lowering drug that decreases serum triglycerides and cholesterol, thereby altering the progression of coronary atherosclerosis. See Principal Investigators (1978, 1984).

confounding factors
The association of a disease and a study factor with a third variable causing a spurious difference between cases and controls. Where an observed association between a factor and a disease is mediated by something else which has not been allowed for.

continuous flow blood cell separator
A system described in 1960 by Dr Jay Freireich. It permits the separation of cells and can be used for plasma exchange, the collection of platelets, and large numbers of lymphocytes for insertion and study of genes. See an interview with Dr Harvey Klein, Chief, Department of Transfusion Medicine at the National Institutes of Health, Bethesda, Maryland, 29 January 1993. Freely available to download at http://aidshistory.nih.gov/transcripts/transcripts/Klein93.pdf (visited 6 December 2005). See also Christie and Tansey (eds) (2003): 60, note 171.

CPIB
See chlorophenoxyisobutyrate.

C-reactive protein
A protein produced by liver cells in response to inflammation and used as a marker of an inflammatory state.

Coons fluorescent antibody method
A technique used for the microscopic identification of native and foreign antigens in tissue sections examined in ultraviolet light and depends on the fact that coupling an antibody with a fluorescent dye does not impair immunological specificity.

deletion
The loss of a piece of DNA from a chromosome that may lead to a disease or abnormality.

delipidation pathway
The metabolic sequence where VLDL is converted to LDL by progressive removal of triglyceride by lipases from the particle.

The process by which fat is removed from lipoproteins during circulation.

diabetes, type 2
An acquired insulin resistance or undersecretion in adult life, usually associated with obesity.

diet–cholesterol–heart hypothesis
Proposes that an excess of saturated fat and cholesterol in food is a *major* cause of coronary heart disease.

diet–heart hypothesis
Proposes that an excess of saturated fat and cholesterol in food is an *essential* cause of coronary heart disease.

dyslipidaemia
Blood fat disorders that favour plaque formation in artery walls, including high triglycerides, low HDL cholesterol and high LDL cholesterol.

edge-irregularity index
A technique applied in quantitative image analysis of coronary angiograms to measure the severity of disease. See Brunt *et al.* (1995).

electrophoresis
A technique using an electrical field to separate a mixture of molecules by their differential migration through a gel or on specially prepared paper.

enzyme assay
A laboratory method to test the activity of an 'enzyme', a protein which has catalytic properties to convert substrate into a product.

factor VII
An essential component of blood clotting (coagulation). A deficiency of factor VII can be congenital, or acquired as a result of liver disease, vitamin K deficiency or other malabsorption conditions.

factorial trial
A randomized controlled trial of two drugs at the same time, which requires four groups: one receives both drugs; the second is given one drug; the third, the other drug; and the fourth receives neither drug (placebo).

familial hypercholesterolaemia (FH)
A genetic disease in which excess cholesterol accumulates in blood and tissues. Plasma cholesterol concentrations may exceed 300mg/dl and even reach 2g/dl.

foam cells
Macrophages loaded with lipid.

free radicals
Molecules with unpaired electrons in the outer orbital resulting in oxidation of other molecules.

Friedewald formula
A method of calculating LDL concentrations when triglycerides

are normal: total cholesterol minus HDL cholesterol minus VLDL cholesterol (estimated as a triglyceride divided by 5). See Friedewald *et al.* (1972).

gas chromatography
A means of separating, identifying and measuring volatile compounds according to how well they move with the flow of a carrier gas, using a fixed solid phase and a moving gaseous phase. Fatty acids separate on columns (celite) containing absorptive material. An inert gas (Argon) is passed through and the fatty acids are detected by ionization.

gemfibrozil
(*Lopid*®, Parke-Davis) A broad-spectrum lipid-modulating agent that decreases serum triglycerides and also lowers LDL-cholesterol and raises HDL-cholesterol.

gene
A fundamental unit of heredity. A locus defines the position of a gene.

gynaecomastia
The enlargement of the male breast.

HDL
See high-density lipoproteins

Hardy–Weinberg equation of population genetics
This equation permits the net effects of evolutionary mechanisms to be analysed and applied to particular populations. It was named for the independent work of the English mathematician Godfrey Hardy and the German physician Wilhelm Weinberg in 1908. Genotype frequencies are given by the equation:

$$p2 \text{ (AA)} + 2pq \text{ (Aa)} + q2 \text{ (aa)} = 1$$

where A and a are two alleles at a gene; p is the frequency of the A allele; q is the frequency of the a allele; $1 = p + q$; $p = 1 - q$.

heterozygous
Possessing two different forms (alleles) of a particular gene, one from each parent.

HMG-CoA reductase [3-hydroxy-3-methylglutaryl coenzyme A]
A fundamental enzyme in the conversion of acetate to cholesterol.

high-density lipoproteins (HDL)
Cholesterol-carrying lipoproteins which may have a protective effect against arterial atheroma.

homozygotes
People who inherit two copies of a defective gene.

homozygous
Possessing identical alleles at a given locus on a chromosome pair.

hypertension
Raised blood pressure.

hypertriglyceridaemia
Raised plasma triglyceride or VLDL concentrations.

intima
The inner membrane of an artery, or a vein. Cholesterol is carried into the intima by plasma low-density lipoprotein (LDL) particles, and plasma high density lipoproteins (HDL) clear it back to the circulation. See www.wri.fi/atherosclerosis.html (visited 8 December 2005).

Lieberman–Burchard reagent
A combination of sulphuric acid and acetic acid that reacts to produce a green colour in the presence of cholesterol. The colour's intensity indicates the amount of cholesterol in solution.

LP receptor
Lipoprotein receptors.

lipoproteins; ß-lipoproteins
Lipid-carrying globulins.

LDL; ß-LDL
See low-density lipoproteins

linoleic acid
An unsaturated fatty acid with 18 carbon atoms and two double bonds (18:2).

lipase
An enzyme normally present in blood and tissues, particularly adipose tissue.

lovastatin
(*Meracor*®, Merck) A statin or an inhibitor of HMG-CoA reductase that reduces cholesterol biosynthesis. Never licensed in the UK. See Appendix 2.

low-density lipoproteins (LDL, ß-LDL)
Cholesterol-rich lipoproteins which, when increased in concentration, may lead to cholesterol deposit in the arterial wall.

meta-analysis
A systematic review of a number of different, but similar, studies using quantitative methods to summarize the results. The meta-analysis pools information to give a large enough sample of sufficient quality and validity to illustrate the results clearly, lessening the effect of random chance. Small, poorly constructed trials with few events are likely to mislead.

Metabolic Syndrome (also known as insulin-resistance syndrome)
People with the Metabolic Syndrome have a cluster of metabolic features, including abdominal obesity; atherogenic dyslipidaemia; elevated blood pressure; insulin resistance or glucose intolerance; a prothrombotic state (having high fibrinogen or plasminogen activator inhibitor-1 in the blood);

a proinflammatory state (having elevated C-reactive protein in the blood). They are at increased risk of coronary heart disease and type 2 diabetes.

microalbuminuria
The appearance of microquantities of albumin in the urine.

myocardial infarction (MI, also heart attack)
The death of cardiac tissue following interruption of the blood, usually caused by obstruction of circulation due to thrombosis in a coronary artery. Infarction can result in permanent damage to an area of the heart.

oestradiol
One of the naturally occurring oestrogens.

oleic acid
A mono-unsaturated fatty acid with 18 carbon atoms and one double bond (18:1). It has a neutral effect on plasma lipoproteins and forms the basis of olive oil.

oxidized LDL
Low-density lipoprotein that has been oxidized. When this occurs in the arterial wall, it accumulates in macrophages.

PAI-1 [plasminogen activator inhibitor type 1]
A prothrombotic enzyme that inhibits the activation of plasminogen by tissue plasminogen inhibitor and thus decreases fibrinolytic activity.

paper chromatography
A technique that separates and identifies pigments and other molecules from extracts that contain a complex mixture of molecules. It relies on the differential affinities of substances for a gas or mobile liquid medium and for a stationary medium through which they pass, such as paper, gelatin or magnesia. Also called absorption chromatography. In paper chromatography the solvent moves up the paper by capillary action carrying along any substance dissolved in it. Once the paper has dried, the individual components can be identified by physical (such as ultraviolet light) or chemical (such as a chemical spray) methods.

phenotype
The observable features of an organism that results from the interaction of genes and the environment.

pleiotropic
Effects that are not anticipated. For example, the pleotropic effects of statins are effects on metabolism that are not directly related to its cholesterol-lowering properties.

polymerase chain reaction
A fast, inexpensive technique for making an unlimited number of copies of any piece of DNA. For the background to this discovery, for which Kary Mullis shared the 1993 Nobel Prize for Chemistry, *see* http://nobelprize.org/chemistry/laureates/1993/mullis-lecture.html (visited 14 December 2005).

pravastatin
(*Lipostat*®, pravastatin sodium, E R Squibb and Sons Ltd) A lipid-lowering compound and a statin which was licensed in the UK in 1990 as a prescription-only medicine.

prothrombotic change
An abnormality in clotting elements in the blood (such as PAI-1 or fibrinogen) that increases the tendency of blood to clot.

remnant particle accumulation
An elevated concentration in the blood of lipoproteins that were triglyceride rich (chylomicrons, VLDL), now partially delipidated, but are resistant to further lipase action. They are remnants of chylomicron or VLDL metabolism that fail to be cleared efficiently, or, in the case of VLDL, fail to be converted to LDL; can cause foam cells and contribution to atherosclerosis as in type III hyperlipoproteinaemia.

scavenger receptor
Receptors on macrophages which take up modified cholesterol.

serum cholesterol
A sterol normally circulating in the blood in the form of LDL (bad cholesterol), HDL (good cholesterol) and to a lesser extent in VLDL.

simvastatin
(*Zocor*®, Merck Sharp and Dohme Ltd) A statin licensed in the UK in 1989 as a prescription-only medicine, and sold over the counter as *Zocor Heart Pro* without a doctor's prescription since 2004.

Southern blotting method
Named after Dr Ed Southern whose invention this was in 1975. A method for detecting the presence of DNA or RNA that permitted the detection, using a radio-labelled probe, of a single copy of a human gene in a sample of DNA fragments separated by size by gel electrophoresis. This involves transfer from a gel to retentive paper (blotting with paper towels facilitates the physical transfer of the nucleic acids).

statins
Inhibitors of HMG-CoA reductase which reduce cholesterol biosynthesis. See also atorvastatin, lovastatin, pravastatin and simvastatin.

stop codon
Any of three mRNA sequences (UGA, UAG, UAA) that do not code for an amino acid and thus signal the end of protein synthesis.

streptozotocin
A nitrosamine compound (specific β-cell cytotoxin) used experimentally in rodents to produce diabetes by destroying pancreatic β islet cells that secrete insulin. It is used clinically for treatment of malignant insulinomas.

Sudan Black
A fat-soluble dye used to stain phospholipids, neutral fats and sterols.

superoxide dismutase
An antioxidant enzyme that converts the free radical superoxide anion, a potentially toxic molecule generated by cells in the body, into hydrogen peroxide.

Svedberg flotation unit (S_f)
A flotation coefficient that describes the gravitation force needed to separate compounds by ultracentrifugation, named after Theodor Svedberg, the inventor of the analytical ultracentrifuge. The flotation rate for a particular lipoprotein species is a physical constant characteristic, after adjustment for concentration effects [1 S_f unit = flotation rate of $1x10^{-13}$cm/s/dyne/gm at 26°C (French (1958): 367)]. See Kyle and Shampo (1997). For human and rabbit ultracentrifugal flotation patterns, see Gofman *et al.* (1952): 121.

triparanol
A cholesterol-lowering agent marketed in the US from 1959. In 1962 the US FDA inspected the manufacturer and discovered that the company had provided falsified laboratory data, suppressing the cataracts that had appeared in rats and dogs receiving the drug, and it was withdrawn from the market in 1962.

tritiate
To label a cell or compound with tritium.

very low-density lipoprotein (VLDL)
A lipid–globulin complex composed mostly of triglyceride and with some cholesterol.

Index: Subject

Index: Names

Biographical notes appear in bold

Key to cover photographs

Front cover, top to bottom

Professor Michael Oliver, Chair

Dr Elspeth Smith

Professor Jerry Morris

Professor Gilbert Thompson

Back cover, top to bottom

Professor Anne Soutar

Professor Sir Stanley Peart, Professor James Scott

Professor Thomas Sanders

Professor John Betteridge

CPSIA information can be obtained at www.ICGtesting.com
Printed in the USA
LVOW051613290512

283769LV00006B/157/A